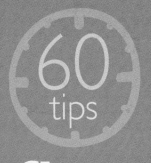

60 tips

flat
stomach

Anne Dufour

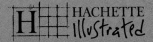

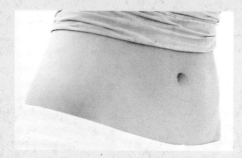

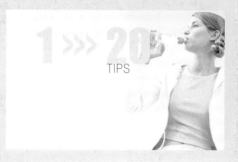

1 >>> 20
TIPS

contents

introduction 4
how to use this book 7
why your stomach isn't flat 8

useful addresses 124
index 125
acknowledgements 126

Note: The information and recommendations given in this book are not intended to be a substitute for medical advice. Consult your doctor before acting on any recommendations given in this book. The authors and publisher disclaim any liability, loss, injury or damage incurred as a consequence, directly or indirectly, of the use and application of the contents of this book.

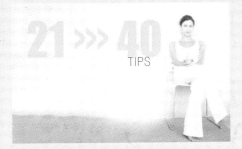

TIPS

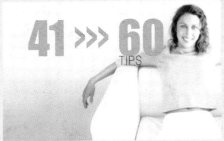

TIPS

introduction

a flat stomach – everyone can have one

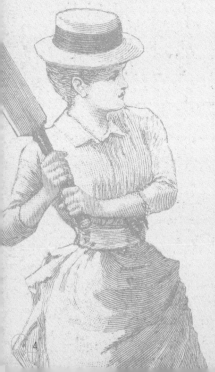

A flat stomach is a fit and healthy stomach. If your tummy isn't flat, it may be because it's suffering, or that your abdominal muscles are not working hard enough.

If it is suffering, it could be because it is malnourished and not digesting properly. It may be that your stomach is unsettled due to hormonal imbalance, stress, adverse reaction to certain medicines or because of an unhealthy lifestyle. Instead of letting your stomach take revenge, give it what it needs: try to stay calm and not get worked up over nothing, breathe correctly during your all-important physical exercise, and pick up a few tips on the side. Sounds fairly straightforward.

So… why is it that such a high percentage of the Western population suffer from so-called 'irritable bowel' or 'spastic colon' syndrome? This condition is characterized by abdominal pain and problems of constipation or diarrhoea, and reacts by the bowel tripling in size.

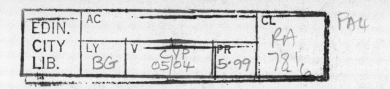
Why is it that 50% of women are unhappy with the appearance of their stomach? The answer is that however simple the theory of a flat tummy, the reality is more complicated. Things are not made easier by the knowledge that our feelings can affect our guts and our tummy may express what our brain is feeling. Neuro-gastroenterologists even refer to it as the 'little brain' and are increasingly looking into its effect on our state of mind. Gastro-enterologists sometimes use low doses of tri-cyclic antidepressants to help with the symptoms of irritable bowel.

What's happening in your stomach?

Moodiness, recurring infections, a creaky back, sleep problems, cellulite, a dull complexion, a lump in the throat – a good number of these woes originate in the gut. We ignore them without even trying to find out why they are happening. Perhaps we would have more respect for our digestive system if we remembered that it is inhabited by nearly 10,000 billion bacteria, mostly in the large bowel, and that it will treat and recycle 60 tons of food and 50,000 litres (88,000 pints) of liquid by the time we die. Most of all, we should remember that if something goes wrong in the little world of our stomach, it is our body as a whole that will suffer. Although we might be eating everything we need, and in the right order, if there are gut problems they will rebound on us later.

The first point: put four-star fuel in your tank and take good care of your gut and the colonies that live there.

Back to the gym tomorrow

Each day, we eat food and draw energy from it. This means that every day an incalculable number of diverse and highly sophisticated actions take place in the body. The digestive and glandular organs involved are the stomach, the small intestine, the colon, the spleen, the pancreas, the liver and the gall bladder. At every meal the miracle is repeated.

It would seem that the least one could do to protect these amazing organs is to keep them inside the skeleton, but no, only our abdominal muscles support these tireless workers. Apart from their function in supporting the internal organs, these muscles work with the diaphragm during respiration. Every time we breathe in the diaphragm descends, pushing down these internal organs and the muscles that support them. If they are not properly looked after, the abdominal muscles lose their capacity to hold in the internal organs, and so the contents of the abdomen tend to fall forward. This is not only unsightly, it is also bad for your back. So, it is vital to look after your body to achieve a flat stomach. There is no easy way to do this. You will have to work to stay in shape and lose those bulges. Remember, the abdominal muscles do not work in isolation – you must make them work. In reality your whole body needs toning up and stimulating. Don't keep putting off buying those trainers: every day that passes is a day lost.

The second point: exercises to strengthen the stomach muscles are a must *and* so is a regular sporting activity for all-over toning.

Waste-treatment blues

Being stressed affects the working of your stomach and guts. You may experience indigestion and heartburn, bloating or abdominal pain, constipation or diarrhoea. In addition the liver and gall bladder are involved in the digestion of fat. When fat enters the first part of the small bowel, it triggers the release of a hormone which causes the gall bladder to contract and release bile acids which act as detergents to make fats more easily absorbed. In particular, too much saturated fat may cause heaviness and bloating which makes you feel under the weather… cue migraines, spots and fatigue. This is the last thing you need for peace of mind.

The third point: give your insides a good clean-out regularly or risk facing the mutiny, strike and resignation of the colon, stomach and the entire digestive system. Time for action!

The stomach and brain are so closely linked that they often communicate without you knowing. You may be suffering from stress to a greater or lesser extent. Remember, your tummy will not be flat until your internal emotional barometer is firmly set to 'sunny' or at least 'changeable'. Contemplate your navel – just this once!

Fighting time

As the years go by, it becomes more and more difficult to stay the course, to maintain your slender figure and to keep off the weight. The time is looming when your hormones will start to fluctuate and a well-managed course of hormone supplements may well be the cornerstone of your success. However, no treatment can ever replace a good daily routine, particularly when you reach your fifties. If you stick to a good fitness routine, it is perfectly possible to stay slim, active and to keep a flat tummy.

how to use this book

This book offers a made-to-measure programme, which will enable you to deal with your own particular problem. It is organized into four sections:

- **A questionnaire** to help you to assess the extent of your problem.
- **The first 20 tips** that will show you how to change your daily life in order to prevent problems and maintain health and fitness.
- **20 slightly more radical tips** that will develop the subject and enable you to cope when problems occur.
- **The final 20 tips** which are intended for more serious cases, when preventative measures and attempted solutions have not worked.

At the end of each section someone with the same problem as you shares his or her experiences.

You can go methodically through the book from tip 1 to 60 putting each piece of advice into practice. Alternatively, you can pick out the recommendations which appear to be best suited to your particular case, or those which fit most easily into your daily routine. Or, finally, you can choose to follow the instructions according to whether you wish to prevent stress problems occurring or cure ones that already exist.

●●● FOR YOUR GUIDANCE

> **A symbol at the bottom of each page will help you to identify the natural solutions available:**

Herbal medicine, aromatherapy, homeopathy, Dr Bach's flower remedies – how natural medicine can help.

Simple exercises – preventing problems by strengthening your body.

Massage and manipulation – how they help to promote well-being.

Healthy eating – all you need to know about the contribution it makes.

Practical tips for your daily life – so that you can prevent instead of having to cure.

Psychology, relaxation, Zen – advice to help you be at peace with yourself and regain serenity..

> **A complete programme that will solve all your health problems. Try it!**

why isn't your stomach flat?

Answer the following statements honestly, ticking box **A**, **B** or **C**, as applicable

You make sure you have breakfast	**A** **B** **C**	every day never sometimes	You have had children	**A** **B** **C**	none one several
You suffer from stomachache	**A** **B** **C**	never rarely often	You are aged between	**A** **B** **C**	20–30 years 30–45 years over 45 years
You snack	**A** **B** **C**	rarely often all day	When you are upset	**A** **B** **C**	you breathe deeply you eat fruit you eat or smoke
You eat mostly	**A** **B** **C**	fresh foods it depends on the day prepared foods	You need to lose a few kilos/pounds	**A** **B** **C**	no just a few yes, a lot
You get indigestion, you feel bloated	**A** **B** **C**	rarely often after every meal			
You sleep	**A** **B** **C**	very well, thank you! OK very badly	If you answered mostly **A**s, you should look at tips **1** to **20**.		
You skip meals	**A** **B** **C**	never occasionally often, as it happens	If you answered mostly **B**s, you should go to tips **21** to **40**.		
You take part in sport	**A** **B** **C**	several times a week sometimes, on holiday never	If you answered mostly **C**s, go straight to tips **41** to **60** – it's time to do something about it!		

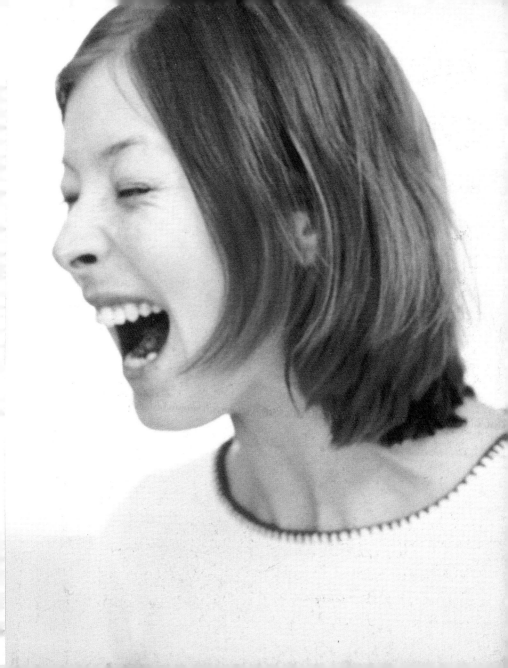

1 ⟩⟩

⟩⟩ Without really knowing why, you've let yourself go recently and it shows in your figure. **Your think your tummy is sticking out a little too much** and it's been a long time since anyone has complimented you on your sporty image.

⟩⟩⟩⟩ **But you don't feel that you've been eating too badly,** or feeling particularly edgy and you don't think you've put on much weight. You don't think it would take too much to get your tummy flat again.

⟩⟩⟩⟩⟩⟩ Don't worry. You're just going through a difficult time! Follow these simple but efficient tips, **and you'll soon get everything back on track.**

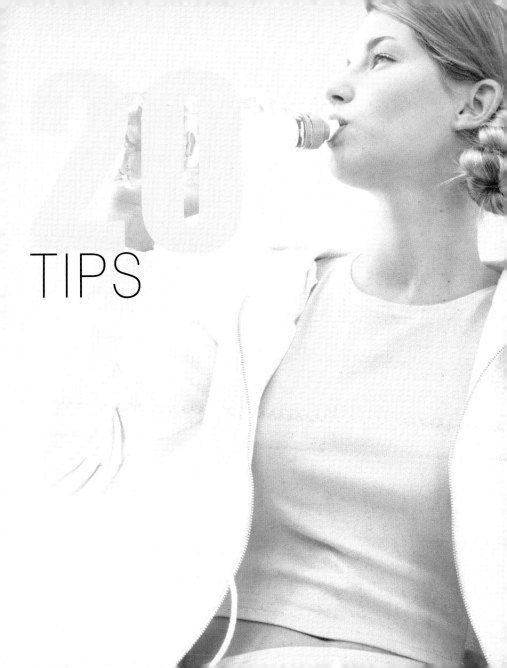

TIPS

01

stand up straight

There were some good things about the deportment lessons of years gone by. Standing up straight and tucking your tummy in certainly does improve your figure. But don't forget to breathe deeply... from the tummy this time!

Posture perfect

Good posture is essential if you don't want your tummy to protrude. It's not just about the way you look either – slouching is also bad for your internal organs and spine. If you want to grow a few centimetres/inches and boast a sporty figure, start by stretching. Hold your head high, look straight ahead... that's all it takes to improve your posture. Good posture means sitting up

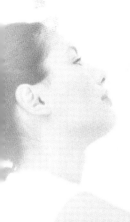

The same applies if your back feels tense after sitting for a long time or if you find it difficult to get up. Do a few quick stretches – this will help you to avoid automatically assuming a bad posture. When you are standing up, imagine that you are hanging from the sky on a thread attached to the top of your head. By pulling your head up, you will straighten up and tuck in your tummy automatically. However, be careful! Don't do this exercise all the time, as it will have a negative impact on your digestion and restrict the depth of your breathing. This would be a great pity, because deep breathing helps stress and can often deflate stomachs bloated from nerves.

straight, your own back against that of the chair to make your stomach muscles work. It's not about flopping down into a soft armchair and slouching.

Head in the clouds

Don't confuse good posture with a straight back. On the contrary, if your back is too rigid, it's because you need to develop the muscles and increase your suppleness.

> The result is that bowel movement improves, you relax and your stomach deflates as if by magic. It's not unusual to drop a skirt size simply by learning how to breathe properly.

> ✳ KEY FACTS

* Your stomach is linked to the rest of your body! Stand up straight and it will lie flatter.

* You need to think about breathing deeply and totally relaxing the stomach.

* Deep breathing can make you go down a dress size!

13 ⓘ

02

The pinch test is, without doubt, the simplest and most effective way of finding out how much excess weight you are carrying, while the effort test reveals the state of your abdominals. Do both without cheating and then test yourself regularly to monitor your progress.

take the test

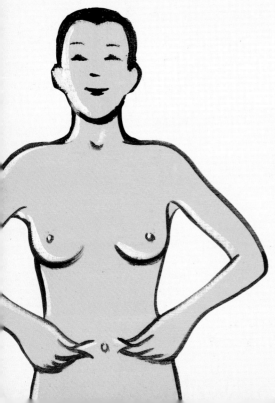

The pinch test

All you have to do is to stand up and pinch the roll of skin under your belly button. If your weight is normal, this roll of skin will be very slight. Sometimes it is even difficult to notice. If you are carrying a little extra weight on your tummy, this roll of flesh gets bigger. If you can only pinch 10 millimetres ($^1/_2$ inch), you should be able to get rid of the roll with regular sporting activity. More than that and you will have to implement an emergency plan comprising exercise, diet and an anti-stress strategy.

The effort test

Just as simple and revealing is this easy test which is performed on the floor. Sit down with your legs stretched out straight in front of you, leaning slightly backwards. Stretch your arms out in front of you while you lift your legs, keeping them straight. Hold this position and time yourself. If you can hold the pose for 25 seconds or more, that's really good! If you can hold it for less than 5 seconds, you've got your work cut out...

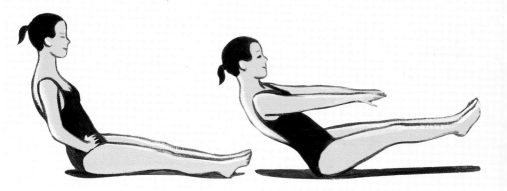

> These tests are essential in determining the condition of your abdominal muscles.

> They also enable you to focus on any slight accumulation of fat, which will disappear all the more easily if you see it as it really is, rather than as you imagine it.

> Take heart: you can't really get to grips with a problem until you know what you are dealing with.

KEY FACTS

* It's important to get an overview of the condition of your abdominal muscles before starting any program.

* It's never too late to work on these muscles.

* It's possible to have weak abdominals and not be overweight, and vice versa.

03

use
chronobiology

Breakfast like a king, lunch like a prince and dine like a pauper. Chronobiology, or recognizing that our body clock governs our internal biology, has become increasingly sophisticated in recent times. We could all incorporate more chronobiology into our lives.

Morning hormones

It's better for your figure to eat more in the morning and less in the evening. This widely acknowledged fact is due to variations in our hormone levels. Whenever you eat, insulin is secreted by the pancreas in order to put sugar and fat into storage, which causes weight gain. In the mornings, however, you are more active and your pancreas secretes

● ● ● DID YOU KNOW?

> Chronobiology is still a little-known area of medicine. It is, in fact, the science of biological rhythms. Biological rhythms are the natural regulators of our daily life, since our internal biological clocks run according to constant, or almost constant, cycles.

> Out of chronobiology came chronotherapy, which is simply the administration of medicines at the right time for the body.

> Tunisian professor, Jaber Danguir, observed Muslims in the run up to

another hormone, known as glucagon, which releases sugar from storage. In the evenings you are less active and insulin secretion predominates, so more of the energy in food gets stored as fat.

Little and often

We now know that dividing our daily intake of food into five or even six meals reduces the risk of putting on weight. It is a case of eating smaller, lighter meals rather than just snacking. In fact, eating small quantities of calories (which may actually take the form of large quantities of food, such as raw vegetables) over several small meals, is not conducive to stockpiling. Breakfast, in fact, is the best time to eat well. If you skip breakfast you may be so hungry mid-morning that you are tempted to eat a high calorie fast-food snack. At midday, you should eat properly, but don't eat fats: this is the worst time for digesting fatty foods.

Ramadan. Despite only eating at night, they still put on weight. This reflects both the quantity they ate as well as the time of day. Other studies have shown that the same meal taken at midday or in the evening has different metabolic consequences.

Dinner should be comprised of proteins (white meat, fish, which are easy to digest) and cereals.

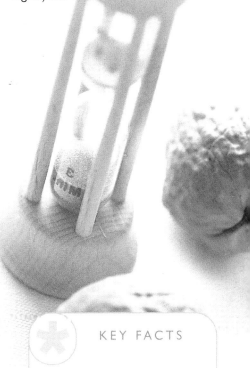

KEY FACTS

* The evenings are the peak time for the secretion of the hormones that store fat.

* It's better to have five small meals than three big ones.

* Have a good breakfast, a low-fat meal at midday and a light meal in the evening.

04 do the dolmen

This very simple exercise helps you learn how to position your stomach correctly. The stomach muscles work non-stop thanks to breathing, so there's no need to warm them up!

Static dolmen Take up the dolmen position – arms and thighs vertical, tummy tucked in, back straight, head and neck extended upwards, looking straight ahead or down. Breathe in, allowing your stomach to relax. Then breathe out and pull your tummy in (always breathe out as you tuck your tummy back in). Count to seven then relax it again. This exercise is easy to do and helps you acquire the reflex of tucking your tummy in.

Right dolmen Take up the starting position. Lock your abdominals then lift and stretch one arm out straight in front. Lower it, then change arms. This exercise will help you to stand up straight. It is more difficult and works the back and abdominal muscles. The 'trembling' of the stomach shows that your abdominals are working. When this trembling becomes generalized, it indicates you should stop.

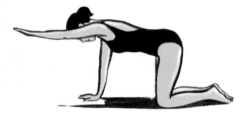

KEY FACTS

* The dolmen should never hurt your back.

* Don't repeat an exercise more than two or three times at first.

05 give up smoking

It is commonly thought that giving up smoking can make you put on weight, but fewer people know that cigarettes are the arch enemy of a flat stomach.

Hypoglycaemia and bad digestion

Smoking is bad for your body for more than one reason. Firstly, it releases the reserves of glucose in the liver, which re-circulates the sugar in the blood. With time this can cause hypoglycaemia and fatigue throughout the entire body. Secondly, it interferes with the digestive juices, particularly when you smoke during or just after a meal. Bloating and flatulence are inevitable. Thirdly, smoking cigarettes is also associated with stomach ulcers.

Give up today! You already know that every cigarette damages your health. Worrying that stopping smoking will make you put on weight is a red herring. Firstly, only one ex-smoker in three puts on weight. Secondly, this is just the body returning to its natural weight so things will be back to normal in 6 months.

● ● ● DID YOU KNOW?

> When you stop smoking, you should avoid certain foods that cause cravings, such as coffee, tea, spices, fizzy drinks (particularly cola) and alcoholic beverages.
> Cut down on your fat and sugar intake as far as possible and you'll keep the weight off
> So, no more excuses – there's no reason for you to put on weight.

KEY FACTS

* Smoking disrupts the digestion and causes hypoglycaemia.

* Giving up cigarettes is one of the most important benefits to your body.

06

choose the right clothes

Your personal style is important. While you are waiting for that ironing-board stomach to appear, choose colours and shapes that hide the protruding bits. Be merciless in throwing out anything that is unflattering or that makes you look fatter or shorter.

No accounting for taste

If you want to hide something, then don't draw attention to it. It's a simple concept. Fashion professionals have always used dark colours, particularly black, and the plainest of fabrics to dress larger women. Today's materials offer a wide range of options for making you 'lose' a few centimetres or inches here and 'gain' a few there. Keep in mind that

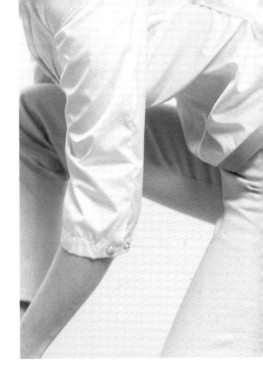

wide shoulders will make your waist look smaller, and matching tops and bottoms will lengthen your silhouette.

No big flowers!

Image consultants recommend that plumper women should choose loose trousers, worn with a long-line jacket without any shoulder pads. If you are big all over, avoid wearing clothes that are too showy with big patterns, flowers or horizontal stripes. Steer clear of any tight-fitting leggings, skirts or dresses, particularly if they are short and/or clinging. You should also avoid wearing belted raincoats, short jackets, two-piece swimsuits, figure-hugging pullovers and T-shirts, trousers and blouses that are fitted at the waist, chunky sweaters, clothes with a colour-change at waist level, very wide trousers and pleated waistbands.

> You can also make the most of your bust by wearing a well-fitting bra and pretty necklines that take attention away from your hips.

KEY FACTS

* Clothes can totally change the way your figure looks. Choose outfits that disguise your tummy.

* The safest bet is still black flowing fabrics.

* Get rid of any clothes that make you look bigger or shorter than you actually are.

07

stay calm

Stress is the number one enemy to beat if you want to lose weight, particularly in the tummy area. Your stomach is your best barometer – if you are stressed, it will be too. And it will stay swollen until you are feeling better!

Stress can make you fat

Some stress is normal and keeps lethargy and apathy at bay. On the other hand, too much will end up tensing the stomach, tying it in knots and, horror of horrors, make you put on weight. Stress affects different people and their stomachs differently – some people lose their appetite and feel full after only a small quantity of food. Other people indulge in comfort eating and crave sugar and fats,

●●● DID YOU KNOW?

> Stress is an insidious and extremely dangerous enemy. It affects the whole body, including the immune system. You have to use all means to fight it; above all, force yourself to get moving to combat the feeling of fatigue that it causes.

> Learn to recognize the signs of stress and diagnose it. Are you aggressive, defensive or depressed? Do you get cravings? Is your workload too heavy? Are you neglecting your hobbies and/or those close to you? Do you have trouble sleeping?

which will be stored in the body as energy reserves. Stress also tends to cause air swallowing and affects the nerve supply of the stomach thus transforming your tummy into a sort of hot-air balloon.

Try Zen

If you are suffering from stress, it's a good idea to keep an eye on what you eat, but it's even more important to get rid of tension. Sign up for a yoga, tai-chi or relaxation course as soon as possible, make sure you get enough sleep, take up a creative activity... but try to calm down... please! Call on the benefits of plants: hops, angelica, camomile, passiflora, lemon balm and lime blossom will have the most benefits. Also, try some essential oils, such as mandarin, verbena, lavender or marjoram, which are excellent calming aids. Use them both at work and at home.

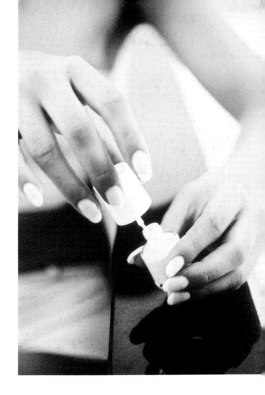

> If you answered yes to one or several of these questions, you should think seriously about changing your approach.

KEY FACTS

* Stress can make you eat: there's no point in dieting if you don't relax.

* Plant extracts, physical exercise or a hobby can all help you to fight stress.

* Stress can make you feel terrible.

08

eat
better

It's simple common sense: when you want to lose weight, you will obviously have to restrict the amount you eat of certain foods. But, above all, you will have to follow some general lifestyle rules. It's the overall view that counts far more than the total calorie content of the food!

Slow sugars and proteins first

Any nutritionist will tell you the same thing, and with good reason: cut back on sugars and fats, eat more slow sugars (complex carbohydrates), fibre and plenty of protein. But you should also think about taking up an 'intestinal comfort' diet. Radically changing what you eat from one day to the next and suddenly ingesting industrial quantities of fibre will make you vulnerable to unheard of levels of bloating, which is just what you were trying to avoid! Make gradual changes, always taking care to opt to eat a little of each food group each day.

Food that's good for you and food that isn't

All light foods are to be looked upon kindly: skimmed (no fat) milk, white fish, poultry, some shellfish, cereals and all fruits and vegetables. The miracle is that these foods are low in calories and very easy to digest. Be extremely wary, on the other hand, of fermented cheese (brie, camembert) or mouldy cheese (Roquefort), fatty meats (pork, lamb, farmed chicken), oily fish (tuna, cooked salmon, herring, mackerel), fried eggs, some shellfish (snails, clams), all prepared dishes (pizza, lasagnes, quiches), very fibrous raw vegetables (introduce them into your diet gradually), oleaginous plants (nuts, almonds), dried vegetables or pulses (except sprouted), green bananas, cooked fats, ice creams and sorbets, the majority of industrially prepared products (stocks, soups, sauces). The list of products that are difficult to digest is very long.

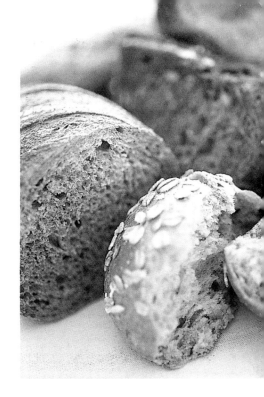

 KEY FACTS

* A low fat diet is also an 'intestinal comfort' diet.

* Don't move instantly from a rich diet to a 100% vegetarian and raw diet.

* Don't be too hard on yourself: don't forbid yourself too many things, just cut back.

Daily life is a huge exercise mat on which you can give your abdominal muscles a quick workout without anyone noticing.

09

try some daily tricks

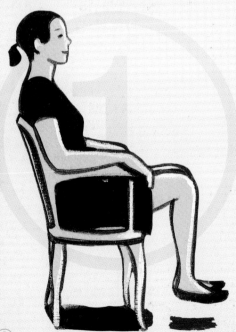

Create your own exercises

Mini-exercises are as efficient as a more traditional session, without the inconvenience of time-consuming classes, because you can do them at the bus stop, while watching television or sitting in a traffic jam. Create your own exercises, depending on your situation. When you're shopping at the supermarket, push on the trolley handle bar, as if pressing it onto the ground, or stop your trolley and try to lift it with one foot while keeping your hands on the bar. Or, alternatively, stand up facing a wall, put your two fists one above the other and push with all your force, as if trying to push the wall over. There's no limit to what you can do.

① In an armchair

Sit down with your back straight, lean your hands on the armrests and lift both your knees at the same time. Count up to seven, relax: count to fourteen and start again. If your abdominal muscles are too weak, you will instinctively limit your effort and lift one knee after the other.

② Waiting for a bus or train

Lift one leg (a few centimetres/inches is enough) and hold the position, locking your abdominal muscles. Try to lift your leg higher and draw circles or letters with your foot.

③ In the car

Sit down with your back straight, tuck in your tummy in the self-stretching position. When you stop, hold out your arms towards the steering wheel and grip it. Gradually lift your knees up to the steering wheel. You can do the same exercise sitting at the table.

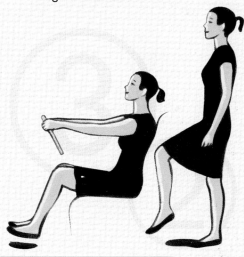

KEY FACTS

* A few mini-exercises each day is more efficient than one session per week.

* Use everything around you to give your abdominals a workout.

* You should soon notice an appreciable improvement in the tone of your abdominal muscle.

10

stop swallowing air

If your tummy is bloated, don't fill it up with more air. Read on to find out what to do and what not to do. You may be surprised to discover that some people swallow air, unaware of the fact that they are doing so.

A dietary culprit

Air is supposed to enter the lungs, not stagnate in the digestive tract. Whether it's aerocoly (an accumulation of gas in the colon), aerophagia (swallowing air) or bloating of the stomach with gas, the cause is nearly always in what you eat. Either you are taking in too much air, or you are eating too much dietary fibre which is broken down and fermented by bacteria in the large bowel.

● ● ● DID YOU KNOW?

> Lots of drinks are responsible for excess air in the digestive system... drinking too much at the dinner table is inadvisable, even if it's just water. Of course, it's much worse to drink fizzy drinks, but sparkling waters are bad too.

> Milkshakes are probably one of the least digestible drinks and certainly the least thirst-quenching.

Gourmets beware!

The delicatessen is full of things that are hard to digest, either because of the food itself or the additives it contains. Factory-made patisserie or cakes, manufactured with low-quality ingredients (hydrogenated fats, additives) should be avoided at all costs. Egg-based mixtures are often very heavy (mayonnaise, ice cream). Even worse are ice cream desserts – remember that cold blocks the digestion. Bear in mind this common sense advice: a convivial meal is food for the mind, but try to listen more and talk less when you are eating, don't breathe in air while sipping a drink that is too hot (such as soup or tea), and most of all, don't chew gum. Not only will you take in air while you are chewing the gum but also, in reaction to the saliva, your stomach will secrete gastric juices for the digestion process, without there being anything to digest.

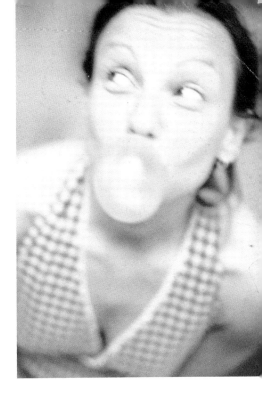

> Most drinks contain digestion inhibitors: additives (cider, beer, syrup, fizzy drinks), tannins (wine, coffee, tea), alcohol (alcoholic drinks), fats (milk, cocoa), refined sugars (all industrially-made sweetened drinks).

 KEY FACTS

* The number one culprit for excess digestive air is you! Rethink your dietary choices.

* Eat calmly and avoid talking too much at the dinner table.

* Watch out for drinks that appear harmless: they may slow down digestion.

11

All vegetables, cereals and other plants have a high complex sugar content. These carbohydrates, which do not taste sugary, should constitute more than 65% of our dietary intake. Rich in a variety of elements, they are valuable allies in the slimming process.

eat complex sugars

Burn the fat!

Complex carbohydrates are found in all fibres. When you eat them you feel full very quickly. They also regulate the appetite by maintaining the secretion of serotonin, important for avoiding severe cravings. Because the sugars in complex carbohydrates are broken down and absorbed more slowly, less insulin is released than by the same calorie intake of soluble sugars such as in cakes, sweets or fizzy drinks, so fewer are stored as fat. In addition, rapidly absorbed soluble sugars cause a rapid rise in blood sugar,

● ● ● D I D   Y O U   K N O W ?

> Not only do complex carbohydrates help you to slim, they also help you to prevent putting back on the weight you have lost... and they make you feel good!

> Complex carbohydrates were once called slow carbohydrates. The name may have changed, but the idea is the same: they pass slowly through the blood, thereby avoiding hypo- and hyperglycaemia and other problems, sometimes even diabetes.

triggering a rise in insulin which, in turn, produces a rapid fall in blood sugar. This fall can be experienced by the body as a craving for sugar. This does not happen with the complex carbohydrates, which are also naturally rich in nutrients (vitamins and minerals) and can lessen the deficiencies commonly found in diets.

Some sugar at every meal

The recipe for eating enough complex carbohydrates is simple: eat fruit and vegetables and/or whole cereals at every meal. You should also reduce your fast sugar intake (sweets, cakes, ice creams) and cut back on all refined products which behave in the same way (pasta, bread and white rice, etc.). Try including lentils and chickpeas in your diet.
Watch your cereal intake at breakfast time. Highly sugared, packet cereals can have the opposite result to the one sought. Read the labels very carefully.

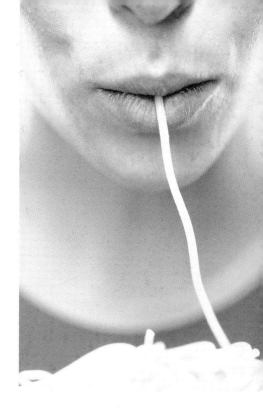

> A diet that is rich in slow carbohydrates is essential in achieving the objective of a flat stomach.

KEY FACTS

* Eat fruit, whole cereals or vegetables at every meal.

* Complex (slow) carbohydrates should constitute more than one half of your diet.

* Banish white sugar and refined products.

12

play sport

For a long time it was thought that sport or exercise alone could not make you lose weight. Now we know that without changing your eating habits, you can shed kilos/pounds in a spectacular fashion... just with physical exercise.

Sport versus the bulge

Sport works on various levels to combat our excess curves: it increases energy expenditure; it mobilizes both sugar and fat reserves; it preserves base energy levels, because muscle mass is not reduced. As an added bonus, it causes an increase in the fat-burning hormones, such as testosterone and the growth hormone, and that's before you even

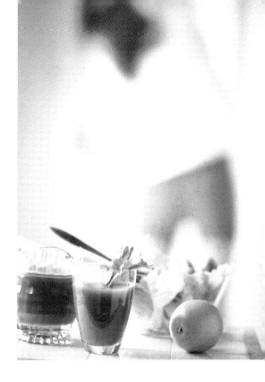

take into account that sport designs and sculpts your body, something that no diet in the world can do. You should consider lifting some weights in addition to your physical activity: you will build some muscle and, while you are sleeping, your body will dip into your calorie reserves to maintain that lean mass.

Get your trainers on!

So, it would seem that physical exercise is a vital part of weight loss, particularly when what you really want is to reshape your figure. Go one better and choose a sport that really gives your abdominal muscles a workout – all dances and dancing, localized weight-lifting, climbing, combat sports or skating. Ideally, you should play sport for at least 30 minutes every day, but a good daily walk, taking care to tuck in those tummy muscles, is a very good start.

> It is impossible to have a sporty figure without doing some sport! Choose an activity that's right for you so that you don't become discouraged after a week, and stick at it. If you can't decide what to do, sign up at a gym.

 KEY FACTS

* Playing sports has nothing but benefits for your health and your looks.

* You have to try to get moving every day for half an hour at a sustained rate.

* Playing sport doesn't let you off doing your specific 'flat tummy' exercises!

13

cook with olive oil

Olive oil may have the same fat content as other oils, but this is the only thing it has in common with them. It should be consumed in preference to all other fats for the delicate stomach and intestines.

Easy to digest

There are fats and there are fats. In general, those present in butter and oils are difficult to digest. Olive oil constitutes a remarkable exception to this rule. Not only is it perfectly digestible, it also facilitates the digestion of other fats, as well as all the heavy foods it often accompanies. Like all fats, olive oil stimulates the contraction of the gall bladder, which pours bile into the duodenum and the small intestine. In this way, it activates the digestion of fats and facilitates the progression of the bolus.

A healthy diet

Olive oil forms a key component of the Mediterranean diet which is thought to be very healthy and beneficial. Drizzling a little olive oil on any dish will add flavour. Raw or cooked, it goes with everything – there are even delicious desserts made with olive oil, a speciality of Provence in southern France. And don't worry about putting on weight: choose a high quality olive oil with a distinctive aroma and flavour so you can use less of it.

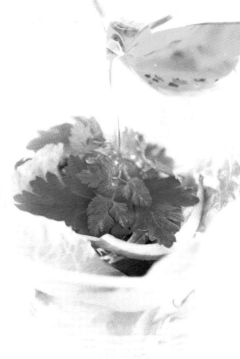

> Furthermore, recent research in the US shows that consuming olive oil regularly doesn't make you put on weight, as long as you don't consume it in great quantities.

 KEY FACTS

* Olive oil is a key constituent of the Mediterranean diet, believed to be very healthy and beneficial.

* Olive oil is thought to aid digestion, combat bloating and ease constipation.

* It's as good on raw food as it is in cooking.

14

less salt, more water

Many people complain of weight gain and bloating and assume that it is due to water retention. You can combat it by eating plenty of vegetables, which are rich in potassium, and restricting your sodium intake. And get moving – literally!

Bloating

Bloating and water retention are typically feminine problems. Stress and a sedentary lifestyle trigger weight gain. Poor circulation causes a sort of internal stagnation, our hormones intermingle and a poor diet doesn't help. Too much salt in our diet may lead to weight gain, high blood pressure and fluid retention. Restart the pump: you need to do some sporting activities, use plants to improve circulation, relax, and above all, change your diet. We eat far too much sodium and not enough potassium – make a move to reverse the trend.

Less salt, more vegetables

Eat less salt. You don't really have to stop adding salt to your food, you just need to avoid factory-made foods. These products represent 96% of our sodium intake and all contain too much salt. Remember, salt is the cheapest flavour enhancer available to manufacturers. Cut back on fast sugars which will cause a loss of magnesium but, on the other hand, eat fresh fruits and vegetables as part of every meal. Don't forget to include fatty acids (omega 3 and 6) which play a role in the balance of body fluids: say hello to oily fish, borage oil and evening primrose oil! Such good habits will help you to avoid feeling bloated and resorting to diuretics.

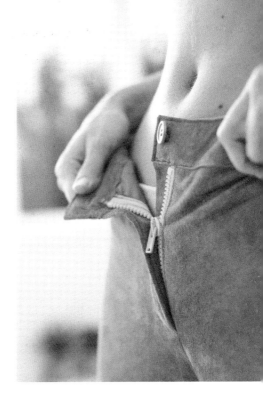

bananas, parsley, spinach, nuts, dates, avocado, garlic, fennel, mushrooms, sorrel, artichokes, broccoli, potatoes (not salty chips!), beetroot and bananas. As a bonus, they are also your best protection from high blood pressure.

KEY FACTS

* An excess of salt will make you bloated.

* Less salt, less stress, more fresh vegetables and omega 3: the best way to keep your figure!

* Avoid diuretics, which are dangerous without good medical reason.

15

eat more fibre

A flat tummy is first and foremost a healthy tummy. One of the key things to do is to add fibre to your daily food intake, in one form or another. If you don't usually eat much fibre, incorporate it into your diet gradually.

Good for your body and zero calories

We should eat around 30 grams (1 ounce) of fibre a day, but the majority of us barely manage a third of that. Fibre is good for transit because it absorbs water, making us eat less, and allows the sugar in the blood to flow more smoothly, so we suffer fewer cravings. All this goodness contains zero calories –

● ● ● DID YOU KNOW?

> Cereals (not packets of breakfast cereals but oats, barley etc.) are the undisputed leaders of the so-called slow sugars. Whole, they also figure among the best sources of fibre, but they are equally rich in precious vitamins B1, B2, B6 and E.

> Get into the habit of eating oatmeal, wholemeal bread, couscous and bulgar wheat. Whole food or health food shops sell less easily available and highly flavoursome varieties, such as millet, barley, buckwheat and rye.

who could ask for anything more? Fibre is absolutely essential for anyone who wants to achieve a lovely flat stomach, but, if you are not used to eating it, it's best to take it easy at first.

Increase the dose

Incorporate fruit and vegetables into your daily diet, and then add whole cereals, such as one or two slices of wholemeal toast at breakfast. Little by little, increase your fibre intake by replacing your usual pasta with wholemeal pasta and brown rice. Top of the list of fruits and vegetables rich in fibre are: broccoli, potatoes (not mash!), carrots, white cabbage, artichokes, dates, dried figs, apples, pears, almonds, avocados, bananas, pineapples and apricots.

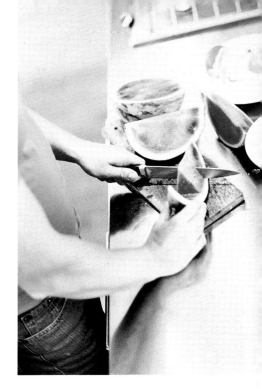

> If you can also add pulses, such as chickpeas, lentils and soya to your diet, you will have an excellent source of protein, which can be easily substituted for meat. It is easy to eat enough of them without resorting to controversial fibre-rich food supplements.

KEY FACTS

* Fibre plays a role in the health, and therefore in the beauty, of your stomach.

* You should eat fibre at every meal.

* Incorporate fibre into your diet gradually. Food supplements are not recommended.

16 replace sugar and synthetic sweeteners

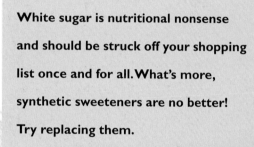

White sugar is nutritional nonsense and should be struck off your shopping list once and for all. What's more, synthetic sweeteners are no better! Try replacing them.

● ● ● DID YOU KNOW?

> Stevia, a plant native to Paraguay is also called the 'sweet herb'. Its sweetening capacity is 300 times higher than white sugar (sucrose).

> In Japan, stevia represents more than 40% of the sweetener market. In the US, it has been used since 1995 as a dietary supplement. However, it is not permitted for sale in the UK or elsewhere within the EU at present, although many people believe it has great health benefits.

White sugar, dark problems

White sugar has many faults and few redeeming features. According to research by the slimming industry, it can easily be replaced with 'synthetic sugar', such as aspartame or polyols, allowing manufacturers to label their products 'sugar-free'. Unfortunately, although these artificial sweeteners do indeed contain fewer calories than sugar, some contain a non-absorbable sugar, so a simple 'sugar-free' chewing gum can make you bloated for several hours... not to mention diet sodas and artificially sweetened yoghurts.

Easy answers

A wide variety of natural sugars is available to sweeten efficiently without any of the drawbacks of these artificial sweeteners. However, they do contain a significant number of calories and cannot be eaten freely: cold-pressed honey, maple syrup, carob (the fruit of the carob tree), stevia (a remarkable plant, at present banned as a food additive in EU countries), kitul (similar to maple syrup), brown sugar and finally fructose. The latter is very similar to white sugar, but with more valuable properties, since its low glycemic index avoids peaks of insulin. With the exception of kitul and stevia, these products are widely available in supermarkets.

KEY FACTS

* White sugar makes you put on weight, some artificial sweeteners are difficult to digest and cause bloating.

* You can replace sugar with small quantities of various natural, flavoursome products.

* Fructose in small quantities can be used to replace white sugar at any time, including in cooking.

> There is an increasingly large body of evidence that the metabolites of aspartame (phenylalanine), found in many soft drinks and manufactured foods, include a number of toxins, and that it is possible to ingest sufficient quantities of these toxins for them to be harmful.

17

Alcohol has few good qualities and a great many drawbacks, the most significant of which is that it is transformed into fat and stored in the tummy area. Do you really want a beer belly?

banish alcohol

Alcohol the troublemaker

If your objective is to lose some weight from your tummy and get rid of your cellulite, then the common denominator is alcohol. Its nutritional qualities are very modest, and its faults far more evident. It is also almost as calorific as fats (7 kcal per g compared to 9 kcal per g). Wine may bring out the flavour of food, but it also tends to cloud our judgement, making us eat more. Beers contain large quantities of carbohydrate and unfortunately stimulate insulin secretion.

● ● ● DID YOU KNOW?

> With regard to health, alcohol is harmful in many different ways. It severely prejudices the digestive system, causes numerous deficiencies in vitamins and minerals (thereby slowing down the functioning of the body as a whole) leading to memory loss and insomnia, and damages the liver causing cirrhosis.

> Obviously, alcohol also affects the nerves and brain. It increases arterial pressure and is bad for the heart. Finally, it predisposes you to cancer, in particular cancer of the larynx, oesophagus, pancreas and stomach.

I'll stop drinking tomorrow…

If stopping drinking is something you really can't contemplate, try to stick to red wine. It is rich in tannins and said to reduce the risk of heart disease (137 kcal per 25 cl). Steer clear of beer (150 kcal per 25cl) and sweet wines (240 kcal per 25 cl) which significantly stimulate the secretion of insulin. In all cases, it's better to drink alcohol during or after a meal, because a full stomach slows down the rate at which it is assimilated by the body. Remember the safe limits of drinking – 2 units per day for women and 3 units per day for men, with some drink-free days each week. Try to cut out aperitifs and drink mineral water with your meal rather than wine. Non-alcoholic lagers are also worth considering, although they are just as high in calories as the real thing. You might also try drinks such as green tea or water flavoured with slices of lemon or other fruits.

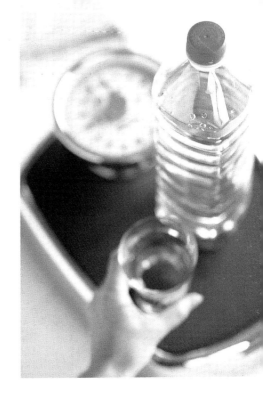

> The right alcohol limit is hard to define, as it depends on the individual. However, 'safe' levels of drinking for women are about a third less than those for men (daily limits are 3 units for men and 2 units for women, where a unit is a glass of wine, a single measure of spirits or half a pint of beer).

KEY FACTS

* Alcohol is bad for your health and your figure.

* Leave behind beer, aperitifs, liqueurs and sweet wines.

* If you want to give yourself a treat, have a glass of a good quality red wine with your meal and really savour it.

18

don't abuse laxatives

All laxatives, including teas, are just for occasional use and should only be used as a last resort. They can lead to a condition known as laxative abuse.

Avoid laxatives

The repeated use of laxatives upsets everything, including the digestive flora. In fact, taking this treatment can cause serious problems, leading to laxative abuse, whereby you need to increase the dose to achieve the same effect. This can trigger inflammation of the colon, various digestive anomalies, kidney problems, potassium loss, toxicity in the liver and really severe constipation when you stop

● ● ● DID YOU KNOW?

> Are you sure you have constipation? Some people naturally visit the bathroom several times a day, whereas others may only do so two or three times a week and, in both cases, this may be normal. If your motions are soft and you can pass them without straining, then you are not constipated.

> Conversely, many people remain constipated for their entire lives, stoutly citing that 'My mother was constipated, and so am I. It's normal.' No, it isn't normal and long-term constipation may even be bad for your health.

taking the treatment. Under the 'avoid' category is paraffin oil, which prevents the absorption of vitamins and minerals.

Take care with plants

The occasional use of gentle, natural laxatives such as mallow or linseed won't do you any harm. Non-absorbed fibres such as bran and frangula can treat constipation effectively – you must take them with plenty of fluids and, in order to avoid wind and bloating, increase the dose slowly. Senna and cascara are harsher and mostly for short-term use and should not be used except in the case of the failure of more general treatments: more physical exercise, eating prunes, fibre-rich foods, water, stress-alleviation, etc. Homeopathy can also help. Some treatments can cause constipation, such as many antacids, antihistamines, diuretics, sedatives, codeine containing painkillers etc.

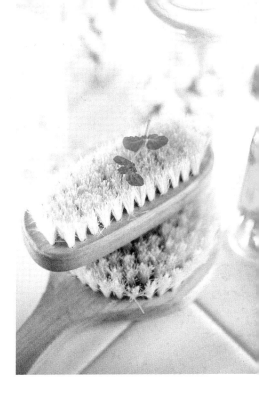

> Even worse, if constipation comes on suddenly and is accompanied by strange symptoms, such as blood in the stools, you should see your doctor in case it is something more serious.

KEY FACTS

* Laxatives should be avoided or only taken occasionally.

* Laxatives are not advised for children, except on medical prescription.

* Prevent constipation with a fibre-rich diet, sufficient liquids and physical exercise.

Charcoal (or carbon) works as a sponge for gas. Completely natural, it is thought to be effective in helping with digestive problems and reducing bloating and flatulence. Take time to learn more about its properties.

19

learn more about charcoal

An ancient remedy

Carbon was used in ancient remedies and is an 'intestinal absorber'. This means that it attracts to its surface the gasses and molecules that have dissolved and been dispersed – nicotine, pollutants, toxins and even some viruses, bacteria and intestinal parasites. It then carries them off in the direction of the 'exit'! What's more, it is thought to be well

● ● ● DID YOU KNOW?

> Vegetable carbon is prepared using specific softwoods, such as poplar, willow, lime or aspen. The wood is burned at high temperatures (700-800°C) without air. The material obtained from this process is steam-treated in order to strengthen its detoxifying properties.

> Studies indicate the efficiency of vegetable carbon in treating digestive disorders, as well as intoxication and even poisoning.

tolerated by the body, causing no bloating or diarrhoea. When used in association with beer yeast (in which case it is called yeast carbon) it is thought to help reconstitute the digestive flora.

Activated charcoal

Activated charcoal tablets are available and may provide relief from gas in the colon. It is thought also to disinfect the colon and combat intestinal mycosis. Carbon has long been blamed for causing constipation and turning the tongue black, both of which have been proved not to be the case. However, it is important that it is not given to children under six years of age.

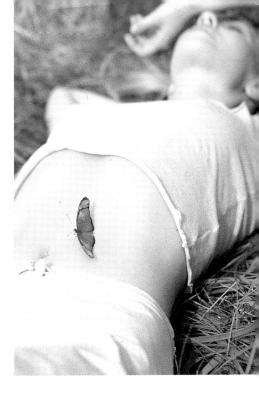

> Vegetable carbon is available in the form of a powder, granules, tablets, capsules and oil capsules.

KEY FACTS

* Vegetable carbon is thought to have remarkable properties for eliminating gas and pollutants.

* It is sometimes recommended for people with digestion problems.

* It must never be given to children under six years of age.

20 think about your medication

Some medication can make you put on weight, and some medicines even encourage you to develop that little tummy that you are going to such great lengths to lose.

The pill and cortisones Some treatments, particularly but not exclusively hormonal ones, can make you put on weight. You can also point a finger at corticosteroids and neuroleptics (drugs used for psychosis) and some hormones. Acarbose, which is used to treat diabetes by slowing down the absorption of sugar, may cause bloating but not weight gain.

Watch your sugar intake The 'side effects' of various medications often fail to appear on the label or in the accompanying leaflet. In general, you should keep a very close eye on sugar content, where the problem principally lies. Avoid all manufactured sugar, choosing fresh fruit instead.

● ● ● DID YOU KNOW?

> As a general rule, sugars, or carbohydrates, contain 4 kilocalories per gram (113 kilocalories per ounce) and are stored as glycogen in the liver and the muscles.
> The body is, moreover, perfectly capable of manufacturing carbohydrate from other nutrients, such as amino acids and fatty acids.

KEY FACTS

∗ Some medicines can make you put on weight – watch what you eat if so.

∗ The watchword is – avoid sugar as much as possible.

case study

«After two pregnancies and years of little physical exercise and a poor diet, I realized that I didn't like my body any more. I wasn't especially fat but my stomach, in particular, was flabby. I decided to get down to some serious sport. I didn't know which one to choose, so I joined a gym near home. I went to see the gym instructor straight away to ask him which equipment I should use to improve muscle tone in my stomach and which exercises I should do at home. He explained everything to me very patiently, helped me to start from the correct position etc. It was great, particularly as I was so 'un-sporty'! I could really see the results after about three weeks. Now, my stomach is firm again, even if it isn't totally flat, and I stand up straighter. I go to the gym twice a week. It's practical and I don't have any excuse not to go. I even give advice to the new arrivals!»

21

>> On one hand, **you feel you're doing all you can to achieve your goal of a 'flat tummy'**, while on the other, the results just don't make the grade.

>>>> If your motivation, good intentions and lifestyle tips haven't done the trick, **perhaps the origin of your problem is a little more complicated.**

>>>>>> While continuing with your exercises, take a new look at the food on your plate. And most importantly, call on nature to give you a boost! **Clay, plants, essential oils, vitamins and minerals may become valuable allies.**

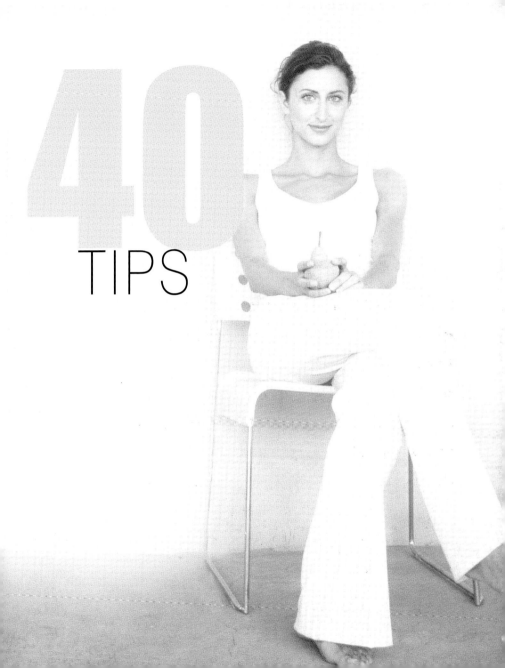

40
TIPS

21

your intestinal flora

There are a few recognized causes of wind and bloating – lactose intolerance, some vegetables like cabbage, onions or some pulses, infections with *giardia lamblia* and it may be worth getting advice from your doctor.

Good guys, bad guys

You simply cannot think about improving your digestion and taking a supplement if your flora is in disarray – and it's easily upset. Stress, antibiotics, too much refined sugar or animal proteins, too little fibre… and pathogenic bacteria will take over. Try to re-establish the balance between the good and bad bacteria in your intestine, otherwise known as the friendly and putrefactive bacteria.

● ● ● DID YOU KNOW?

> The digestive system is home to more than 100,000 billion bacteria of hundreds of species. Some are beneficial (acidophilus, bifidobacteria) and others are not (strepto-cocci, coliforms, anaerobes).

> If you weighed all the bacteria in your body, they would weigh about the same as your liver.

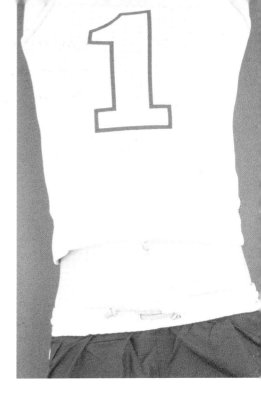

Plan of attack

To protect your precious flora some advise eating high-quality yoghurts (homemade is generally thought to be best), fermented milk or, strangely enough, sauerkraut. Some people suggest more drastic measures and propose a 'fermentation treatment' with up to as many 5 billion bacteria in each dose. If you are susceptible to diarrhoea, start with a half dose at the beginning. These products are live and, if you opt for the dried format (powder, tablets), they usually need storing in a cool place.

> The bacteria fulfil multiple functions: some synthesize vitamin K but essentially they break down dietary fibre etc.

 KEY FACTS

* Balanced intestinal flora is vital for good health.

* The balance depends on the predominance of good bacteria over bad.

* There are more bacteria in the average gut than cells in the whole body.

22

be wary of dairy!

Milk and dairy products are often the cause of flatulence, digestive discomfort and diarrhoea – not at all compatible with a nice, flat stomach! Cut out dairy products and see if there's any change.

Lactose intolerance

When you think of the foods that trigger digestive problems and cause gas, top of the list are dried beans, onions, wheat and apple juice. Milk, however, should also figure high on the list of culprits. Doctors and patients are becoming increasingly aware of milk intolerance. It is not normal for adults of any species to drink milk, let alone milk of another species. As infants, virtually all of us have

●●● DID YOU KNOW?

> Dairy products are a good source of calcium and you can reduce associated saturated fats by avoiding butter and cream and using skimmed milk (no fat milk) and low fat dairy products.

> Good sources are yoghurts, fermented milks and goats' or sheep's cheese.

> Additionally, good quality calcium can be found elsewhere, such as canned sardines and mackerel with bones, almonds, cabbage, mineral water rich in calcium, dried figs, tofu, dried beans, chickpeas, etc.

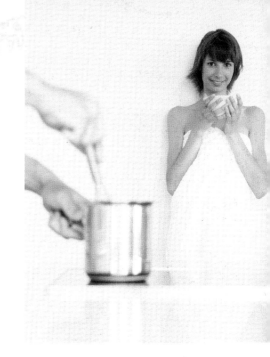

the enzyme in the wall of our intestine that breaks down lactose, the sugar in milk, to simple sugars. After infancy, many of us, especially people from the Mediterranean, Africa and Asia, stop making lactose and this means that when we drink milk unabsorbed lactose passes into the large bowel where it is fermented by the gut flora and causes problems. The symptoms mostly take the form of simple bloating or loose stools but very occasionally, symptoms may be more severe. Cut out dairy products completely in order to see if your digestive symptoms disappear.

Two notable exceptions

Only yoghurts and milk chocolate sidestep this ban. In the case of the former, the ferments 'predigest' the lactose for you, whereas in the case of the second, the cocoa is thought to stimulate the enzymatic activity and increases the efficiency of the lactase (the enzyme that digests the lactose). You can easily replace most dairy products with their equivalents made with soya, almond or rice milk.

KEY FACTS

* Milk and dairy products can lead to digestive problems.

* Yoghurts and milk chocolate are usually not the culprits.

* Replace cow's milk with vegetable milks, which are healthier and more digestible but if you can't give up milk you can buy lactose tablets over the counter.

23

save your skin

Variations in weight are bad for the skin in the stomach area, which tends to stretch and tighten up again at the dictate of those extra kilos/pounds. Caring for this skin is vital if you want a smooth, taut stomach.

Winner of the beauty product of the year award: olive oil

Over the course of time and with constant dieting, the skin of your stomach loses its elasticity. If in addition to this it is poorly moisturized, it will give in to the flab to a greater or lesser extent. Don't listen to the claims of all the manufacturers of (sometimes very expensive) slimming creams, but think about using olive oil on your skin every

● ● ● DID YOU KNOW?

> Body creams designed for mature skins are formulated according to the same principle as anti-wrinkle creams. They boast moisturizing, firming and anti-ageing properties.

> Remember: if you choose this type of product or a course of essential oils, the action is as important as the care. You have to massage every day, and not just on the tummy, the thighs and buttocks too.

day, a product that moisturizes, firms and combats oedema. Remember too, that the best beauty products are still a balanced diet, particularly one that's rich in good fatty acids (olive oil) and in vitamins (fresh fruits and vegetables).

Slimming creams:
a course of treatment

Firming cosmetic products containing natural ingredients, such as essential oils, are best. If your problem is cellulite, you should know that caffeine-based creams really do fight the fatty deposits, particularly if their formula includes a vein tonic (horse chestnut, hamamelis). The essential oils which are also efficient are Atlas cedar, lemon eucalyptus, sage and rosemary. Mixed with a vegetable oil (olive, borage, evening primrose) and applied daily, they are thought to help stop the tissues from becoming overloaded.

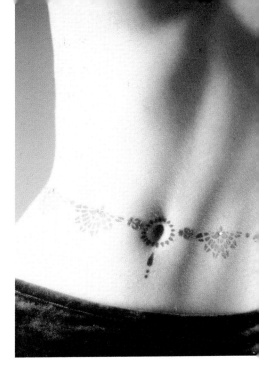

> As often as possible, rub your skin in the shower with a loofah mitt, to activate the circulation as a whole and, horrible but extremely efficient, end your shower with a jet of cold water from your toes up at least as far as your knees.

KEY FACTS

* Extra kilos/pounds make the skin around the stomach area rather delicate.

* Moisturizing and firming products should be applied every day: try essential oils.

* Activating the circulation makes 'flat stomach' cosmetics more effective.

24 try essential oils

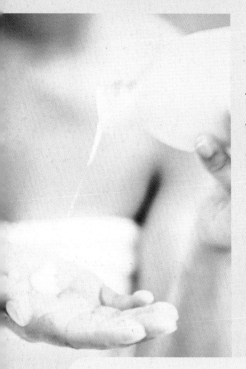

The principal cause of bloating, flatulence and other digestive disorders is a diet that is either unbalanced or too rich. Essential oils are a good choice of treatment to help you get rid of the problems linked to the accumulation of gas in the intestine.

●●● DID YOU KNOW?

> Essential oils should be used with caution. Do not exceed the advised dose and, above all, *never* ingest pure essential oil.

> Always mix essential oils with a vegetable oil, milk or honey. They mix very badly with water and could become toxic for the liver if not correctly used. Choose biological products where possible.

Ginger, lavender
and peppered mint

Essential oils are like guiding spirits. If selected with care and used correctly, they are extremely powerful. To help you achieve your goal of a flat stomach, think about adding the following essential oils to your alternative medicine cabinet: camomile, ginger, lavender, peppered mint and juniper. Used in conjunction, these essences can be even more efficient in accelerating the digestion, dispersing gas and generally refreshing the stomach.

Essential oils:
how to use them

Essential oils can be for internal or external use. In a glass, mix a tablespoon of top-quality honey with a drop of peppered mint or ginger essential oil then fill

the glass with hot water and sip slowly. Similarly, you can have a digestive massage. Mix 1 tablespoon of vegetable oil (grape seed oil is best) with a drop of juniper and mint essential oils. Warm the preparation a little over boiling water and use to massage the stomach area, ideally in a clockwise direction. If pregnant, research the essential oils that are safe to use.

> Take care: essential oils are photosensitive. If you use them for a stomach massage, do not expose that area to the sun for 12 hours afterwards, to avoid blotches on the skin.

KEY FACTS

* Essential oils of camomile, ginger, lavender, peppered mint and juniper are digestives.

* Prepare yourself an anti-bloating mix whenever you feel the need.

* Do not exceed the doses and follow the instructions for use of the essences.

25

get on that mat

Exercises on your back really give your stomach muscles a workout. They are also the most efficient! This exercise is particularly good for flattening the stomach. Always take care not to hurt your back.

Suffer for beauty

The following exercise should not make your back hurt at all. Protect your back by lying completely flat with all your vertebrae touching the ground. If you're a bit out of practice and haven't taken much physical exercise recently, it is better to soften your back up a little over the course of the first few sessions before doing the exercise properly.
On the other hand, don't worry if your thighs hurt a little – this is normal.

Also, when working on your stomach, you should feel it tremble slightly; never put your hands under your bottom to support the pelvis; stop immediately if you feel pain in your back. If you are in the wrong position you risk getting sciatica or lumbago.

Stretch out, but don't fall asleep!

Lie down on your back, hands behind your head and legs bent. Sit up gently, unfurling your back, one vertebra after the other and exhaling deeply. This exercise is more difficult the closer your feet are to your bottom. If you are not on your own, ask someone to hold down your feet. Avoid pulling on the nape of the neck with your hands.

Start with a few repetitions but aim to repeat the lifting movement 40 times, breathing regularly. The rhythm should be constant, and there is no need to relax the stomach muscles when letting your head back down or to rest between each lift.

● ● ● DID YOU KNOW?

> Do this exercise in the evening. The so-called 'static gymnastics' just warm up the body and do not stop you from sleeping.

> Don't rush – do the movements slowly and persevere.

> If you are feeling extremely motivated, you could also do this alternative exercise: stand up, legs together and straight, bend down and touch your feet with the ends of your fingers. Stand up fully each time.

KEY FACTS

* Do the exercises, lying down, at the end of your session (after the dolmen, for example, see Tip 4).

* The fitter among you can start straight away with the mat exercises.

26

pay a visit to your gynaecologist

The stomach is the centre of femininity. It is also a sensitive seat of emotions, both good and bad, as well as being a part of the body where hormones can go wild.

Girl talk

If you think your stomach is too large, but you are not overweight and you don't have any digestive problems, consider booking an appointment with your gynaecologist. Some gynaecological problems such as an enlarged womb due to fibroids, ovarian cysts or endometriosis can give rise to bloating, frequency of micturition (the need to pass water often) or painful or heavy periods, and

●●● DID YOU KNOW?

> When you have your period, you feel as if you have put on weight. In fact, not only is this a temporary feeling, what you really acquire is volume rather than weight. And your stomach can get quite large.

> The drop in progesterone, a female hormone, favours the retention of water in the tissues and can cause constipation. As a result of hormones, the lower stomach is also congested and cannot tolerate being cramped.

the appropriate treatment can be extremely helpful.

Borage or evening primrose oil

Obviously, if you have a gynaecological disorder, you should consult your doctor. If your problem is simply pre-menstrual syndrome, you should be able to control this problem or eliminate it altogether. First of all, restrict your salt consumption. Then, every month take a course of borage oil or evening primrose capsules. These oils, rich in fatty omega 6 acids, are anti-inflammatory and can help with painful periods. Some women find that applying a natural progesterone cream to the stomach area also works well. If this does not work for you, it may be worth seeing your doctor. The oral contraceptive and some anti-depressants can also help pre-menstrual syndrome.

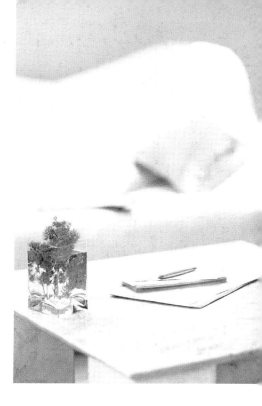

> Add to this the fact that tiredness can increase the feeling of heaviness and that the digestive system itself can be affected by this hormonal upheaval. Things soon get back to normal (until the next month!).

KEY FACTS

* A gynaecological disorder could be the cause of a large stomach. Visit your doctor if you are in doubt.

* If you have pre-menstrual syndrome, take evening primrose or borage oil, or apply some natural progesterone cream.

Baths can be really good for both body and soul. Hydrotherapy, or water treatments, can be invigorating, relaxing or slimming, depending on the type of water into which you blissfully sink.

27

sink into a relaxing bath

Cleopatra's time-out

Bathing cleanses, softens and refreshes the skin, relaxing and stimulating it. It also relaxes the muscles and the mind and is ideal for soothing stomachs that are bloated with stress and anxiety. If you want to lose weight, choose algae and/or essential oils of geranium, sage or rosemary for their stimulating effect.

● ● ● DID YOU KNOW?

> The heat of the bath dilates the pores and facilitates the penetration of active ingredients. Choose your essential oil according to the effect you wish to achieve.

> Circulation: cypress or sandalwood (there are oils available that combine red vine and hamamelis). Firmer skin: eucalyptus, pine, rosemary. Relaxation for a good night's sleep: bergamot, lavender, orange, verbena.

Hydrotherapy: instructions for use

First of all, find a little time for yourself – 'me time' – and head for the bathroom. Run a bath at a temperature somewhere between 30 and 37°C (86 and 99°F) and pour in some slimming essential oils – such as lemon – mixed with a vegetable oil such as sweet almond. Enjoy this time of peace and relaxation – make it a weekly event. You might want to investigate other relaxation aids for the bath, such as a plastic mattress for the bottom of the bath or a bath pillow for your neck. These are very affordable and are really worthwhile as they make the bath more relaxing and increase the efficiency of plants and essential oils. Remember, too, that you also breathe in the essences you put in the bath in the form of water vapour, so the scent of the oil is also important.

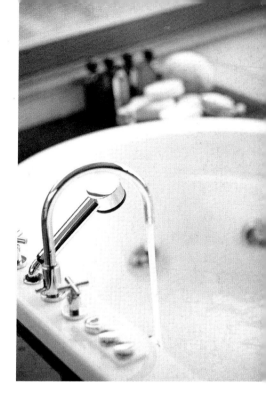

Stimulation: pine, rosemary, sage, savory. Troubled skin: elder, lime-blossom and camomile (prepare an infusion, strain and add to the bath); you can also put some brown rice in a square of gauze, leave the sachet to soak in the water and use it to rub your skin.

KEY FACTS

* Choose the essential oil according to the effect you are seeking: stimulation, relaxation, slimming, etc.

* Always mix essential oils with two tablespoons of milk, sweet almond oil or olive oil before adding them to your bath.

28 take an anti-stress cure

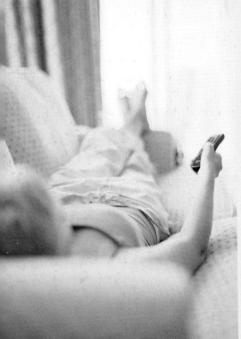

Don't let stress get you down. It will upset everything you do, and your figure too. Take natural food supplements to help combat stress: a useful aid for when it becomes too entrenched.

No stress

Stress unbalances different hormonal systems and some people who comfort-eat may put on weight. We also now know that stress devours vitamins and minerals, leaving a body suffering from deficiencies: a body that, all of a sudden, doesn't work properly. Stress is a plunderer of vitamin B, magnesium and calcium in particular. Stocking up the body on micronutrients will make stress lose its grip, and the body will relax, letting go of both its aggression and its kilos/pounds. If stress is upsetting your sleep pattern, you should consider using one of the various sedative plants.

Shock treatment

Here's an efficient treatment: 1 or 2 multivitamin tablets (according to the dosage) and minerals morning and evening, plus a vitamin B complex three times per day, plus 2 to 4 capsules of marine magnesium, plus 1 gram (0.035 oz) of calcium per day and some vitamin C if not already present in your multivitamins. Some complexes contain all of the above and you must read the labels carefully to avoid overdosage. If you suffer from mild to moderate depression St John's wort may be helpful but it does interact with several remedies and you should always take advice from your pharmacist or doctor. You should also consider the plants that can help you to get gradually back on track. Ginseng for example is an 'adaptogen' and thought to help you to adapt to new situations.

KEY FACTS

* Stress harms your health and affects your weight.

* In cases of stress, there's no point in putting yourself on a diet which is stressful in itself. Deal with the cause of the stress.

* Vitamin B, magnesium and calcium should be your first recourse.

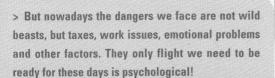

> But nowadays the dangers we face are not wild beasts, but taxes, work issues, emotional problems and other factors. They only flight we need to be ready for these days is psychological!

29 have a cup of green tea

Green tea is one of Nature's miracles: not only is it a really healthy drink, it may also help you to lose weight. Add it to your arsenal of 'flat stomach' weapons straight away.

Triple action: mechanical, mental and chemical Tea is rich in theine, thought to accelerate the burning of stored calories. Flavenoids, in turn, play an additional role in this phenomenon and speed up urinary elimination. Green tea also stimulates the movement of the intestine, combating constipation, and its polyphenols benefit the digestive flora, essential for good digestion. Finally, green tea calms agitated minds, eliminating the thought that obsesses all those who suffer from constipation – going to the bathroom.

Join the tea-drinkers club! Around 14,000 cups of tea are drunk every second. It's the most widely consumed drink in the world after water. Sign up to the tea-drinking club and give your body the three or four cups of green tea per day that it deserves. You will find it at most supermarkets. However, keep in mind that tea contains caffeine which is a mild stimulant, so care should be taken. If you tend towards insomnia, don't drink it after 3pm.

● ● ● DID YOU KNOW?

> Green and black tea come from the same plant. The difference lies in the manufacturing process.
> Green tea is simply heated, whereas black tea undergoes various treatments (drying, chopping, fermentation, etc.), which diminishes its beneficial properties.

KEY FACTS

* Green tea can act as an aid to slimming.

* It stimulates digestion, is relaxing and improves the digestive flora.

30 cook with herbs

Herbs are reputed to facilitate digestion. Make them regular guests at your dinner table, add their lively flavours to both raw food and cooked dishes, and let them brighten up your meals in a flash!

A mine of vitamins Cooking with fresh herbs will do nothing but good for your figure. These herbs add zest and flavour to your dishes, and so reduce the need for so much fat and salt. They are also tremendous sources of nutrients, minerals and vitamins in particular. And most of all, they help digestion.

Fresh or nothing Sprinkle dill on your tomato salad, oregano on your pizza, rosemary on grilled food, savory on vegetables or a few chives in your omelette. Aromatic herbs can be used on all occasions and in all meals. They are at their best by far when fresh. If you can't get fresh, use frozen – dried herbs have lost a large part of their goodness. You might also try preparing some fresh herb tea to drink after you have eaten. Dill and mint are particularly good for this, and they give off a wonderful aroma!

KEY FACTS

∗ Cooking with herbs is healthy and a good habit to acquire if you want to lose weight.

∗ Some herbs can really help you combat bloating.

∗ Choose fresh (or frozen) herbs rather than the dried variety.

No, vitamin C is not just a cold cure!

It also plays a key role in the body functions

that are important when you're on a diet.

31

replenish stocks of vitamin C

Top of the vitamin chart

Vitamin C (ascorbic acid) is a simple sugar and powerful reducing agent. It is essential for the synthesis of collagen and wound healing, the synthesis of haemoglobin in red cells and is found in high concentrations in the adrenal gland. It also plays a part in resisting stress. All in all, vitamin C makes your body work faster, harder and really makes you feel like exercising.

● ● ● DID YOU KNOW?

> It is better to get your vitamin C by eating a healthy diet, but if you find it impossible to do this, you should try natural or synthetic vitamin C.

> With natural vitamin C supplements (e.g. acerola or dog rose) you also get the goodness of more esculosides (circulatory vitamin elements), vitamin P (bioflavenoids: an anti-oxidant and venous tonic), calcium, trace elements and pectin (fibre).

A full tank of vitamin C

Vitamin C is found in abundance in fresh fruit and vegetables but is easily lost in cooking water and by boiling. Eat around five portions of fresh vegetables every day and not only will you lose weight, you will also have a tank full of vitamins. Stress and illness increase daily requirements, so do ensure you are getting enough vitamin C. Take vitamin C in combination with tyrosine: these two nutrients complement each other perfectly (see Tip 50).

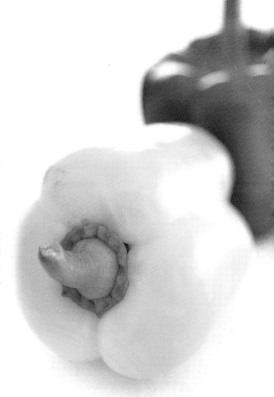

> Natural vitamin C penetrates the cells more efficiently, because it is released more slowly. Vitamin C does not make you jittery, so you can even drink it in the evening.

 KEY FACTS

* Vitamin C is essential if you want to lose weight and find the energy to get moving.

* Vitamin C is to be found in fresh fruit and vegetables.

* In the form of a food supplement, choose natural vitamin C over its synthetic form.

32

give homeopathy a try

Extremely good at combating all functional symptoms, homeopathy is an efficient medicine that is not only gentle on the body but effective at tackling bloating, particularly if you have a nervous disposition.

Diagnosis

Bloating is, in the vast majority of cases, a functional problem. In other words, it is not due to damage to an organ but rather to a problem with the way that the organ functions. The remedy for almost immediate relief will depend on where the signs or associated symptoms are located. The correct diagnosis is vital, and it may be the case that there are several homeopathic remedies.

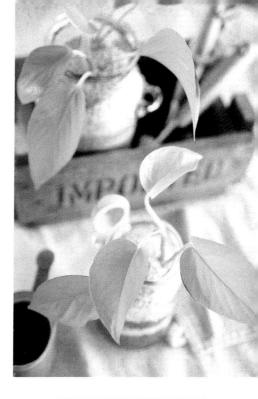

Nux vomica or Valerian

If your bloating is confined to your stomach, with a feeling of constriction and an improvement when you burp, try *Carbo vegetabilis*. *Lycopodium* will relieve bloating from the lower part of the stomach, with some relief by passing wind. *Nux vomica* targets after-dinner lethargy. Bloating due to nerves responds well to Valerian and, when the cause is your period, try *Cocculus indicus*. All these remedies should be taken in a dose of three granules three times a day in 9C.

> That doesn't mean that homeopathy is just a placebo, but rather that the granules only work within a very specific framework, in the same way as a key fits a lock.

 KEY FACTS

* To gain instant relief, find the right anti-bloating remedy for you.

* There are many books available on homeopathy. Research the subject further.

* The remedy that suits a friend or relative may not necessarily be the right one for you – learn to listen to your needs.

33

You can make your shower time a real part
of your flat stomach program. And if you can
get hold of a massage shower, the effect will
be ten times better!

change your
shower

Cold water treatment

There is more to splashing yourself with water than you might think. It's not just about getting out of bed and diving into the shower before getting ready for the day. Water improves the way your body works, but its effectiveness depends upon the temperature of the water and the products used. Cold water tones the skin, firms the tissues and boosts circulation. Hot water gets rid of muscle spasms

●●● DID YOU KNOW?

> The so-called 'Scottish shower', alternating hot and cold water, causes the blood to flow to the surface of the skin – tone and vitality is guaranteed. This type of shower may even reduce fatigue and slow down the ageing process.

> It is thought to be able to strengthen the immune system and thereby can prevent infections and boost the body's 'mechanics', improving the digestion, stimulating the circulation, making you feel more active.

and relaxes you. With a new showerhead you can give yourself proper massages on the thighs, stomach and buttocks. Be brave: the cold water on your feet and legs is really good for you, even if it comes as a bit of a shock at first.

The right temperature

The important thing in the shower is the temperature. It can often be too hot: above 38°C (100°F) it makes you weaker, puts stress on your heart and hinders good blood circulation. Water around 30°C (86°F) is the ideal temperature to make you feel good (and comfortable!). Between 24°C and 30°C (45°F and 86°F) the shower will refresh and tone. Avoid using shower gels, except those of a very high quality, and avoid aggressive shower gels followed by moisturizing lotion, which dermatologists say is bad for you. Instead, choose soap-free bars or gentle soaps that are not so harsh on your skin.

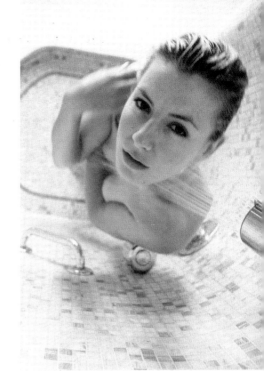

> If you want to make the most of your shower, give yourself a friction rub once a week with a loofah mitt or flannel: you will get rid of dead skin cells, have a really good anti-cellulite massage and possibly lose a few centimetres or an inch or two from your tummy!

KEY FACTS

* Showers can be very good as part of your flat stomach program: cold water and friction rubs are recommended.

* Avoid shower gels that dry the skin.

* The 'Scottish shower' can fight the ageing process.

34

increase your serotonin levels

Sugar addicts know all about serotonin levels, if not by name then by the effects. After eating sugar, they feel better, even calmer, but the repercussions of sweet treats inevitably gather around the tummy. How can you limit your consumption of sweets without making yourself nervous and irritable?

Serotonin: a passport to serenity

Why are we so drawn to sugary foods, particularly when we feel worried or are about to have our period? They trigger the secretion of serotonin, a calming substance produced by the brain to combat stress. So, you really can get addicted to sugar if you consume three

> Half the Western world is on a diet at any one time. Unfortunately dieters usually cut out foods rich in tryptophan, all too often linked to fat. The result is a drop in plasmatic tryptophan levels and, therefore, in serotonin, which leads to a deterioration in mood and memory and an increase in cravings.

> Fast sugars make you fat, particularly in the case of women suffering from stress, those affected by premenstrual syndrome or seasonal affective disorder (see Tip 59) or those who have given up smoking (nicotine increases serotonin).

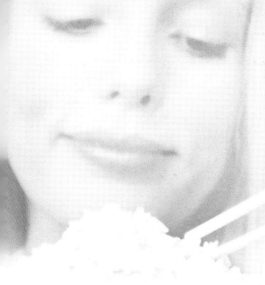

to six sugar-laden meals a day. The plan is to deal first with the nerves and achieve a calm state of mind, conducive to concentration, without eating too much sugar. How do we achieve this high level of serotonin? The answer lies in eating foods that are rich in tryptophan and in 5-hydroxytryptophan, precursors of serotonin.

> An excess of sugary foods in the diet is also linked to an increased risk of obesity and heart problems.

Eat yourself thin

The first part of the plan involves replacing fast sugars with foods that have a low glycemic index, such as brown rice, dried beans or lentils. The second is to incorporate into our daily diet natural foods that are rich in serotonin precursors, such as eggs, soya, tomatoes, aubergines/eggplants, avocados, wholemeal bread, dates, nuts, prunes. The third is not to overlook omega 3 fatty acids, which aid the action of the serotonin at cell level and are found in rapeseed oil or nuts and in fatty fish (mackerel, sardines, herring and salmon).

KEY FACTS

* When you eat sugar, you secrete serotonin.

* Produce serotonin without putting on weight by eating foods rich in tryptophan, omega 3 and fatty acids.

* Nicotine increases serotonin levels: when you give up smoking, you crave sugar.

35 eat chilli!

If you don't put chilli in your food, perhaps you should rethink your dietary habits. Chilli (hot peppers) can help you lose weight. Read on to find out how.

Chilli eats sugar Capsaicin, the principal ingredient in hot pepper, stimulates the production of adrenaline and nor-adrenaline which allows you to burn sugars and fat deposits. Pepper, particularly red pepper, is effective on this level, as well. Pepper improves digestion and decongests you when you have a cold to boot! How many of you knew that?

Fire alarm If you don't usually eat chilli, go steady at first. Of course it does set your mouth and your senses aflame, but it's all in a good cause. Consider using it to liven up your cooking. You could prepare a hot chilli oil yourself, by marinating fresh chillies in the bottom of a bottle of olive oil. Don't go too far, though, as chilli can irritate your digestive system, particularly in the anal region. It is not recommended for anyone with an ulcer, those with clotting problems or those who are prescribed anti-coagulants. It is also not recommended for women who are pregnant or breastfeeding.

●●● DID YOU KNOW?

> Capsaicin is thought to combat the formation of blood clots and to relieve a number of inflammatory disorders. It is also said to protect the stomach from the effects of alcohol, aspirin and acids and even thought to have anti-carcinogenic properties.

KEY FACTS

* Chilli pepper can help accelerate weight loss.

* Hot peppers should always be used with caution, because they can irritate the nervous system.

36 trust in plants

Digestive teas are back in fashion. As they become increasingly widely available in supermarkets, cafés and restaurants, their positive properties are now being recognized. They can help with flatulence, slow digestion and the resulting bulging tummy.

Plants help with your digestion Mint, fennel, hyssop, oregano and anise are some of the plants that can help dispel gas from the intestines. They are known as 'carminatives', which means that they can accelerate digestion. It is often their essential oil that is active, hence their pleasant and fresh aftertaste in the mouth.

Long live herbal tea! For flatulence, the French herbalist M-A Mulot advises the following combination: 15g anise, 5g caraway, 5g coriander, 10g fennel, 5g cumin, 10g mint, 10g Melissa, 15g costmary, 10g lime blossom, 10g orange blossom, 10g verbena. Have this mixture prepared at the pharmacy and leave one tablespoon to infuse in $\frac{1}{2}$ litre (1 pint) of simmering water. Drink shortly after you have eaten. (NB 10g=$\frac{1}{3}$ oz).

KEY FACTS

* Try to replace your after-dinner coffee with a cup of herbal tea.

* Mint, verbena or anise should be incorporated into all diets to aid the digestion process.

79

37

try chromium

Chromium won't make your stomach melt away, but by improving the use of the sugar you do eat, it will limit the amount stored. If you don't have a particularly sweet tooth, go straight to the next tip.

Sugar and the cells

The original property of chromium is that it can improve the sensitivity of the cells to insulin. Sugar can then penetrate these cells more easily, spending less time in the bloodstream as a result. It regulates sugar levels in the blood for 24 hours after absorption. Chromium is of real value in the prevention and treatment of diabetes, but in a more general

●●● DID YOU KNOW?

> Even though some studies have shown that chromium actually makes you lose weight, it is best just to make it a part of the battle against the bulge, which is enough in itself.

> Due to the improvement by chromium of the manufacture of serotonin, a chemical messenger that curbs your hunger pangs, it is a valuable ally on a diet.

way it helps control sugar for those who find it difficult to regulate their blood sugar levels.

One tablet every morning

Chromium is found in liver, egg yolk, thyme, wholemeal cereals, seafood, meat and beer yeast. Refined (white) sugar and flour no longer contain chromium and our levels of this mineral are usually low. 1kg (2lbs) of whole wheat contains 175 micrograms, whereas after the refining process, this content is reduced to 23 micrograms. Make sure that you are getting enough chromium by taking one 200mg tablet every morning. There are various products available on the market. Since the body absorbs this mineral slowly, it is best to buy it as picolinate or nicotinate in order to reap the full benefit of its properties.

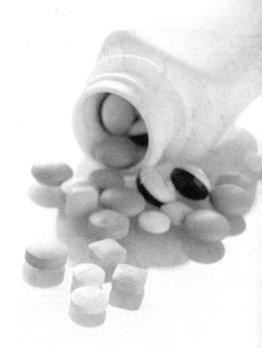

> Not only is chromium essential for the metabolism of carbohydrates, it also reduces cholesterol levels and protects the arteries. There are no obvious signs of deficiency, but people who play a lot of sport, diabetics and those with a sweet tooth may need more in their diet.

KEY FACTS

* Chromium improves the use of sugar, reducing our craving for sweet things.

* Chromium tablets can be bought at pharmacies or health food shops.

* Regular courses of treatment will not have any side effects.

38

enjoy a massage

There's nothing like a good massage to relax you and your stomach. Your tummy can sometimes get tied up in knots or blow up like a balloon up just to get the care and attention it needs. Massage or self-massage can help deflate the problem, quite literally!

Circulation and massage

Massage makes the stomach more supple, getting it moving the way it should. It can also rid you of bloating, constipation, flatulence and other tensions, as well as boosting flagging circulation, thereby assisting the fight against excess fat. And don't forget that it also gets your muscles ready for a workout – do it both before and after exercise to avoid aches and pains.

Our skin is a great fan of massage. Every centimetre/inch of the skin is packed with nerves and vessels, which can be awakened by massage. Massage improves the circulation of blood and lymph, and it helps remove other waste. It has an impact on the whole body.

Take care, literally

Self-massage is a little gift you can give your tummy every day. Standing upright, put your warm, flat hand on your abdomen. Massage slowly in a clockwise direction (in the natural direction of the digestive process), using a regular motion and rhythm. One or two minutes is usually enough, but you may benefit from longer, remembering to breathe slowly and deeply. This simple movement enables you to improve the operation of your digestive system, calms irritations of the stomach and restores balance to the nervous system.

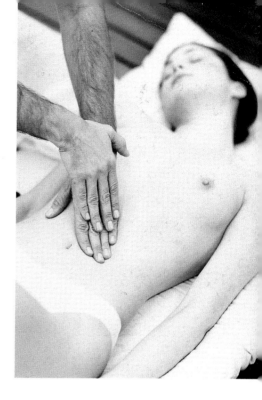

> Try to give yourself a daily massage lying on your bed, just before dropping off to sleep. This action will help the digestive system to do its job more quickly.

KEY FACTS

* Massage re-establishes harmony for a Zen spirit and a flat tummy.

* Massage your stomach in a clockwise motion to ease digestion.

* Self-massage is a simple, everyday solution.

39 experiment with clay

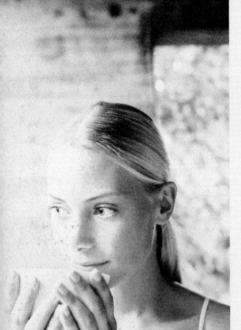

Bloating is invariably due to excess gas. There is nothing like clay for absorbing this gas, and it has the added bonus of carrying away toxins en route. It also eases pains caused by colitis.

● ● ● DID YOU KNOW?

> If you get colitis with severe inflammation, consider combining your internal treatment with clay poultices, but always consult your doctor before embarking on any treatment.

> Prepare a thick paste or use a ready-made product that needs to be warmed, not over direct heat or in the microwave, but just by adding hot water or wrapping it in cloth and pressing it against a hot-water bottle.

An all-purpose cleaner

Clay makes a highly effective natural absorbent and adsorbent. Rich in minerals, this special substance attracts gases to its surface and impregnates itself with these gases, freeing you of them. Outside and in, clay works relentlessly to absorb, cleanse, regenerate and heal. And while it does that, it also makes your complexion fresher and your skin more beautiful.

A glass of milk is good for you!

Clay can be prepared easily by mixing clay powder and water (mineral water, if possible). The resulting drink is called 'clay milk' and, a three-week course, with one glass before every midday meal, gives excellent results. If the way it looks puts you off, you can always opt for clay capsules or tablets, but remember to drink plenty of water. If you get colitis,

drink your clay in the morning, on an empty stomach, in order to capture the poisons and rebalance your still unsettled intestinal flora. If you are on any medication, ensure that you take it separately from the clay, or the clay might end up absorbing the medicine. In any case, check with your doctor or pharmacist to find out if there are any possible interactions between the clay and your medication.

KEY FACTS

* Clay has extraordinary properties for absorbing gas and deflating the stomach.

* A clay treatment should last a minimum of three weeks to one month, even several months in the case of long-standing colitis.

* Always take clay treatment at a different time to any medicine, and increase the dosage progressively. Check with your doctor or pharmacist if there are any interactions between your medication and the clay.

> Apply this directly to the painful area. The poultice needs to be really thick. Applied two or three time per day over the course of a month, you will soon notice that the pain starts to fade or even disappear.

40 cook up a storm

Learning to cook involves not only choosing the ingredients but also about cooking methods. Steaming and braising can help bring you nearer your goal of a flat stomach, while fry-ups will only set you back several steps.

Casseroling, steaming and stir-frying

Eating good, healthy food is all well and good, but you can spoil it with inappropriate cooking methods. The principle is to cook food for as short a time as possible and at the lowest heat possible. The aim is to produce food that is flavoursome, high in vitamins, easily digested and low in calories.

Take care with your cooking methods

Steam partly eliminates the fat in foods and preserves the vitamins and minerals, so try using a steamer. Grills all too often char food, so you should always remove the blackened part, which is unhealthy and highly indigestible. The microwave oven retains the vitamins but transforms the proteins, so is not recommended for milk and meat. Cooking with a conventional oven is fine, as long as the temperature is not set too high.

● ● ● DID YOU KNOW?

> Even if it says so in the recipe, never salt the water when you start cooking. Through osmosis, the salted water is thought to draw the mineral salts out of the vegetable.
> Neither should you add bicarbonate of soda (sodium bicarbonate) to the cooking water. This might keep the lovely green colour of vegetables, but it destroys the vitamin C.

KEY FACTS

* The cooking method is as important as the food itself.

* Steaming is a simple way of cooking, and one of the healthiest.

case study

I've stopped fighting myself.

« My mother is of Mediterranean descent, and so am I. We're plump, it's written in our genes! Over the years, I've fought to get rid of my fat. I put myself on draconian diets, depriving myself even of raw food and vegetables. The more I went on, the bigger my stomach became. Until, that is, I went to see an endocrinologist, who explained it all to me. He told me that fat was intelligent tissue, which had multiple functions in the body and the more I deprived myself of it, the more my body would avenge itself by storing fat. He re-educated my eating habits, teaching me to eat according to my hormonal profile. I was really surprised because I was allowed to eat sugary foods, meat and a little bit of everything I wanted. Most of all, he encouraged me to take up sport. In fact, by eating a lot more and getting a little bit more exercise, things got better. Now, I've lost my extra weight, I'm still on the plump side but I can't do anything about that, and my husband likes me the way I am. I don't have to wear shapeless clothes anymore – I can wear the latest fashions. That changes everything! »

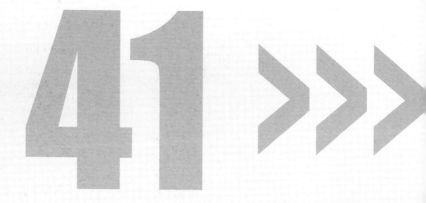

41 »»

» Do you think yours is a desperate case? That your tummy gets bigger every day and **whatever you try nothing seems to work?** You're almost certainly not on the right path to tummy-tackling.

»»» If the problem is hormonal, you need to gently re-establish the balance. **Waste no time in seeking the advice of a sports specialist,** or give yourself a massage to boost your system: sometimes, you need to ask for help!

»»» The following pages contain original ideas for **helping you to achieve the figure of your dreams.** Try them before resorting to extreme measures, such as plastic surgery.

60
TIPS

41

consult a nutritionist

Do you find it difficult to eat properly? Or has it all been going on for too long for you to be able to sort it out on your own? A consultation with a nutritionist is a good idea if you feel that you are not in control of what goes onto your plate.

A food specialist

A nutritionist is a food expert. He or she will understand the impact the food you eat has upon you. This is important because it's not just about eating less in order to take in fewer calories. It's about eating better and more healthily. We all know people who can eat whatever they like without putting on so much as a gram or ounce, while others get fatter just looking at a lettuce leaf… this might

● ● ● DID YOU KNOW?

> Your food notebook is not about punishment: there's no point in hiding things to avoid a reproving glance from the nutritionist. The objective is for you to consider your binges (if you have them) not as faults, but as situations that require resolving.

> The notebook can't make you lose weight, of course. However, noting down what you eat does mean that you can measure and understand the issues.

sometimes depend on your genes or hormonal profile. The nutritionist should be able to give advice on all aspects. This help will be invaluable if you have tried and failed on a whole range of different diets of all types and your body is stuck on 'storage'.

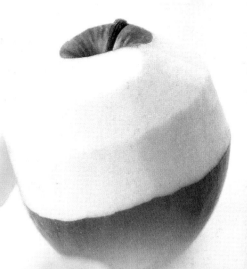

Oh, so you're supposed to write those peanuts down too…

The first thing a nutritionist will ask you to do is to write down in a notebook everything you eat. And that means absolutely everything, including those few peanuts, that little glass of wine and the nibble of your colleague's croissant! At the end of the first week alone this notebook will give you a clearer idea of how much you eat as opposed to how much you think you eat (there's often quite a difference) For instance, does it all look reasonably acceptable, or do you realize that you spend all day snacking?

Are all the food groups present in sufficient quantity? Does your diet balance out over a day or a week, or perhaps not at all? As a practical exercise, take a notebook and divide a page into three columns headed: Where and when? Why? How much? Fill it in as you go along. The nutritionist will interpret your notes and be able to give you valuable advice and foodback

> It's also important to keep this private food diary for a reasonable period of time, so that you can study all the facets of your food behaviour.

KEY FACTS

* A nutritionist will help you adapt your diet to your body and your personality.

* Keep a food diary so that you can keep track of what you actually eat.

42 make time for yourself

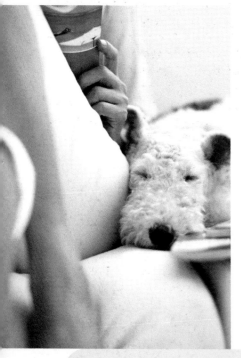

If you want your flat tummy back, you need to equip yourself with the necessary resources. You need to devote some time to achieving your goal – you can't expect your stomach to change unless you're prepared to make a few changes yourself!

> Force yourself to reconsider yourself as a human being worthy of interest, and take care of your body in general and your stomach in particular. It's up to you to take the first step if you want everything to change for the better.

Leave the cares of the world behind

If you can't set aside half an hour during the day to do your exercises or take a relaxing bath, it's because something isn't right in your life. Of course we all have to work, look after the house, wash, sleep, spend time with friends or children (or both), lend a listening ear to others, but it's easy to forget yourself in the middle of all this. You have to realize that you can only take care of yourself by freeing up time from other activities, possibly to their detriment. Try to stop worrying about the rest of the world for a little while. If you can't do this, or if you think that an hour spent on yourself is a waste of time, then it may be the right moment to ask yourself a few questions about where your life is heading. The truth is, you are mistreating your body and it is paying you back by swelling up and plaguing you with cravings.

Look after yourself

Start by making the decision and telling those around you: every evening, at such and such a time, I don't want to be disturbed. Often, your nearest and dearest will perfectly well understand this need and leave you alone to spend time in the bathroom or taking a calming walk. Let yourself go and unwind in the bath, massage your feet, go for a walk at sunset, write a personal diary – all these activities will enable you to really relax and become aware of your own existence and needs.

KEY FACTS

∗ Take the time to think about yourself.

∗ Set aside at least half an hour during or at the end of the day, just for yourself.

∗ Take care of your body if you don't want it to wreak its revenge.

> The first thing to do is to spend some time on yourself. Perhaps you'd rather slump in front of the television than unwind in a bath or lie on your bed. That's a mistake! Remind yourself of a valuable piece of psychology: 'a tyrannized body will soon turn tyrant'.

43

check out caffeine

What if drinking coffee (without sugar of course) could make you thin? To a degree it is true but be careful, as the caffeine it contains is no harmless substance.

Too much of a good thing…

Caffeine increases the calories you use up while you rest. It activates the production of heat and with it the combustion of calories. With the occasional exception, our body is at rest for most of the time, and in these conditions it burns around 1 calorie per minute but, under the influence of caffeine, this is increased by up to 10% for the hours following a cup of coffee. That's not bad when you add it up! Significant research has been carried out on this subject, but there is a problem. It appears that if, on

> In some countries, pharmacies stock a coffee product enriched with guarana and chromium (see Tip 37), making a caffeine concentrate. Beware of the not inconsiderable side effects: anxiety, insomnia, palpitations, diarrhoea, heartburn, etc., and find your own personal tolerance level.

> You can also try asking your chemist to prepare caffeine capsules if you don't like the taste of coffee. If you do this, don't exceed 150 milligrams of caffeine per day (equivalent to two and a half cups of coffee).

average, you drink more than five cups of coffee per day, the effect is reversed. So do bear that in mind.

Lose weight while you sleep

Drinking too much coffee will not help you lose weight while sleeping due to the alerting effects of caffeine. Obviously you can only achieve a flat stomach by combining an appropriate diet with regular exercise. But consider this: simply drinking coffee or tea increases the amount of calories you burn. The effect is not highly significant which is why caffeine is not licensed as a weight-reducing agent but drinking coffee is pleasurable, without the cost of extra calories. Foods that contain caffeine include coffee, tea, guarana, maté, chocolate and cola. Don't add sugar or you will lose all the benefit of the caffeine. Watch your coffee intake if you suffer from migraines, have a heart condition or are diabetic, pregnant or breastfeeding.

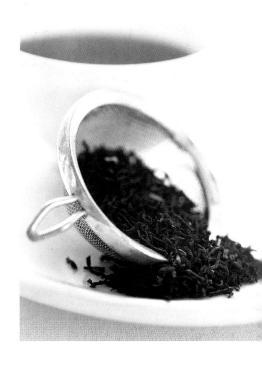

> With regards to slimming creams that contain caffeine, it appears that they do not have the same drawbacks but may be less effective. The active ingredient works topically and does not get into the bloodstream. You can even buy tights that contain it, in micro-drops set in the fibre!

KEY FACTS

* Caffeine increases the amount of calories you use while you are at rest.

* It is highly active but there are side effects if you are susceptible.

* Slimming creams containing caffeine may offer benefits without side effects.

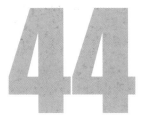

44

stimulate your muscles

Equipment that stimulates your muscles can be a useful aid in your physical exercise program. It can't work miracles, but it will help tone your abdominal muscles, for example when they have been misshapen by pregnancy.

You have to suffer to be beautiful

Electro-stimulation is, as its name indicates, the electrical stimulation of the muscles. Although the objective is to develop them, in reality it enables the muscles not to melt away like snow in the sun. Even for a minimum efficiency, however, the intensity of the current must be fairly high – athletes who use this type of equipment really suffer, under the watchful eye of their trainer!

● ● ● DID YOU KNOW?

> Some people confuse electro-stimulation with electro-lipolysis. The latter, which is the breaking down of fat, has nothing to do with muscular stimulation, and involves sticking needles into the skin. It is not available in all countries, so do some research.

> Driven by a small motor, the electro-lipolysis needles give out impulses that dislodge fat in the adipocytes. This type of treatment is normally painless and the improvement is apparent, as long as the electro-lipolysis is adapted to your needs.

The frequency of the current varies between 50 and 70 hertz, and the time of the contractions between 1 and 5 seconds. Well-managed sessions can give excellent results in achieving a toned stomach, for example, after a pregnancy. You need to follow the advice of a qualified practitioner – don't just try this out on your own. The main value of this equipment is that it works on the muscles that are difficult to reach in physical exercise. Find out if it is available in your country or area.

High-quality equipment

You should invest in high-quality equipment or the results may not live up to your expectations. It may sound silly, but you need the sticky pads that attach the electrodes to your skin to still be sticky after five sessions. It is important to seek the advice of any physiotherapist before buying equipment like this – get him or

her to tell you exactly where to place the electrodes, which need to be positioned correctly on the muscular insertions. Never use electro-stimulation equipment on a damaged muscle or if you have a pacemaker.

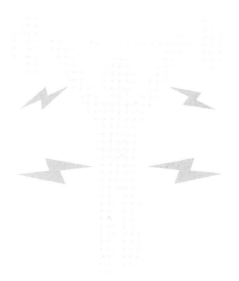

> Whatever technique you use, if you don't work on the causes, the consequences will reappear quickly, and you will regain the weight in no time.

KEY FACTS

* Seek the advice of a physiotherapist before using electro-stimulation equipment.

* To get results, you must invest in high-quality equipment.

45

push those
pedals

Pedalling is great for working your abdominal muscles. Remember how it used to make us suffer in gym classes at school. Take it up again and pay a little more attention this time than you did as a reluctant schoolchild. Pedal power works!

Better results than real cycling!

Pedalling is probably the most efficient of all exercises, as well as being one of the easiest. Separate each movement: breathe in as you stretch your legs, breathe out as you bring them back up. Breathing is particularly important in this exercise. Tuck your tummy well in as you breathe out. You can do the same exercise pedalling backwards. Why? No reason, it's just very fashionable! Funnily enough, cycling on a real bicycle doesn't work your abdominals in the same way.

Pedal for your stomach

Lie flat on your back, hands behind your head, knees bent, feet on the ground. Pedal in series of about twenty repetitions, keeping you tummy tucked in all the time. At the end of the exercise, bring your feet and legs up onto your body and rest your feet. If you can't do the exercise without lifting your back off the ground, lift your legs. The higher the feet, the easier the exercise, but remember, the harder it is, the more effective it will be!

The scissors

The scissors – does that ring any bells? Begin with the same starting position, but instead of pedalling, stretch your legs out straight ahead then cross and uncross them to each side, and up and down. As with the pedalling, start high and come down as low as possible without your back leaving the floor. This exercise is efficient but is also difficult to measure. Ideally, you should finish with your legs horizontal without hurting your back.

● ● ● DID YOU KNOW?

> Unfortunately, the most efficient abdominal exercises tend to be the ones that make you suffer!

> If you feel in good form, increase the degree of difficulty. For example, make little figures of eight with your feet instead of just pedalling.

> Most importantly, concentrate on doing the movements correctly or you will risk tiring yourself out, gaining no benefit and hurting your back into the bargain.

KEY FACTS

* Put some effort into it. To get the best results, really go for it!

* Make sure you do a minimum of 20 repetitions.

46 unblock the hara

There's a lot to be learnt from Chinese medicine. The hara is the area situated below the tummy button, which needs unblocking in order for energy to circulate.

The laughing hara The hara is well known to those with an interest in Chinese medicine and those who practise the martial arts. Located just below the navel, it represents the centre of the body where the energy (Chi) is concentrated. When the hara gets knotted, the stomach swells and rebels, and energy is prevented from circulating. When this happens, you will really feel the bad effects. Unblocking the hara is most important.

Contemplate your navel Qi Gong includes a specific exercise for establishing a dialogue with your hara. Just sit on the edge of a chair, back straight, eyes closed, knees apart, feet flat on the ground. Place your left hand on your thighs, palm outwards, then place the right hand on top, palm inwards. Breathe in and out very slowly and deeply. Imagine a cloudless sky while you concentrate on your navel until you start to get a warm feeling.

● ● ● DID YOU KNOW?

> Qi Gong is based on the theory of acupuncture. Anyone can do it, regardless of age or physical condition.

> It is absolutely essential to synchronize your postures and your breathing. The word Qi elsewhere means breath and air.

KEY FACTS

∗ In Chinese medicine, when the hara becomes knotted, all energy is blocked.

∗ A simple Qi Gong exercise can get the energy flowing once more.

47 investigate thalassotherapy

There's nothing like a thalasso treatment to boost your morale and slim your tummy! Trust in the sea and fill up on iodine, restore your inner calm and discover new ideas about healthy, slimming food.

Real therapy With thalasso, the base metabolism is increased by iodine. It has a diuretic effect and calms digestive problems. Also, the individual care and just walking in the sea increases the return of blood to the heart, boosts the circulation and flushes the system. The anti-retention effect is guaranteed!

A special treat Enjoy a week (or at least a few days) of thalassotherapy, popular in France but becoming increasingly more so worldwide. You can focus on slimming, circulation or stress, depending on your problems. The combination of the bubbling water (massages the body and stimulates the digestion), jet shower (firms and improves circulation), seaweed wrap and sweating (promotes the elimination of toxins through the skin) and water aerobics (combines the effects of exercise and abdominals) is really revitalizing.

● ● ● DID YOU KNOW?

> Thalasso treatment offers a combination of benefits. Apart from the seawater there are other elements to consider.

> Algae is packed with vitamins and minerals, while sea air carries a variety of beneficial substances in aerosol form.

KEY FACTS

∗ A thalasso treatment renews and revitalizes you deep-down.

∗ Seawater, algae and sea air come to work together to get you back in form.

∗ If possible, treat yourself to a week of thalossotherapy.

48

take a look at reflexology

The solar plexus gets blocked when you suffer stress or tension. By using the reflexology points on the palm of your hand and the soles of your feet, you can relax and set your energies flowing properly again.

Get the right reflex

When you suffer from stress, blocked energy can coil up in the abdominal region, slowing digestion and stiffening the stomach. The reflex zones that correspond to the abdomen are found in the hand and are easy to stimulate, but you should also think about massaging the soles of your feet. This simple action releases the accumulated tension which can translate into a bloated and painful stomach. The plexus point, when correctly pressed, will release your solar plexus, while the colon region point will stimulate your digestion. Whenever you hit on a sensitive, painful or weak point, reduce the pressure.

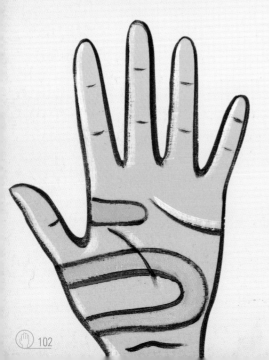

Plexus and colon: the same battle

Start by sitting yourself down as comfortably as possible in a calm, relaxing place. Look for the reflex points on your palm that correspond to the plexus (in the case of stress) or the colon (in the case of problematic digestion), or even both if necessary. Work over the whole of your palm, then find the specific spots, pressing slightly harder. You may feel a little discomfort, which should start to ease as the massage continues. For the feet, take hold of the toes in your left hand, pressing the reflex zone of the solar plexus with the right hand. Make clockwise circular motions on the spot.

KEY FACTS

* Establish a routine for massaging your sensitive reflex zones.

* Some discomfort is normal: it should stop quickly.

49

splash out on a skipping rope

There's never been anything better than a skipping rope for working all the muscles in your body, and you can do this when you want and where you want. If you think that's funny, remember that it is a real sport, and try skipping for just 30 seconds running.

Skip the right way

Skipping increases your heart rate, develops the muscles in your legs and forearms, improves balance, breathing and motor coordination, and works the abdominals. A skipping rope is an ideal piece of exercise equipment, but use it intelligently. Start by buying the right length rope for your size: it should brush the ground from hip level when you hold the handles with your elbows pressed against your sides. Never skip rope unless you are wearing properly cushioned footwear.

A real training program

Warm up by walking or running on the spot for a few minutes. If you have not used a skipping rope for exercise before, start by skipping from one foot to the other on tiptoe (not on your heels). Then, feet together, knees slightly bent, jump up and down, but not too high. Build it up gradually, starting by alternating steady jumping and rest periods of equal length. You should be able to do 100 jumps without getting out of breath, then 60 to 70 jumps per minute for 2 to 3 minutes. If all goes well, you should be able to link up several series of jumps and then gradually increase the number of jumps per minute. Always stretch your legs at the end of a session while you are still warm to avoid stiffness.

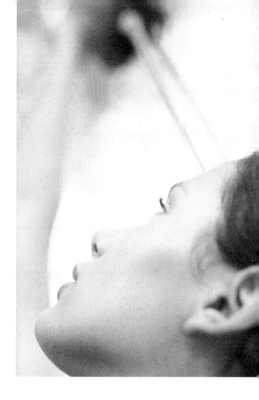

> Using the skipping rope is a demanding exercise. If you haven't played any sport for a long time, get in shape first of all by walking. If you have a heart condition, seek the advice of your doctor before starting any intensive program.

KEY FACTS

* Skipping with a rope gives your abdominal muscles a workout.

* Start by taking slow jumps interspersed with long rest periods.

* Always make sure that you wear well-cushioned shoes to protect your joints.

50

take tyrosine

If you are depressed or if stress is making you overeat, tyrosine can calm you down and stop you storing your stress-calories on your tummy.

Fat reshuffle

Tyrosine is an amino acid, one of the building blocks of proteins in the body. It is an essential ingredient in the manufacture of two hormones – thyroxine from the thyroid gland and adrenaline from the adrenal gland – as well as dopamine and nor-adrenaline which are neuro-transmitters found in the brain. Thyroxine and adrenaline speed up the body's metabolism and nor-adrenaline

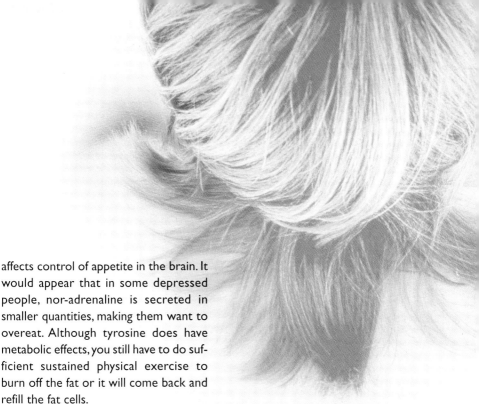

affects control of appetite in the brain. It would appear that in some depressed people, nor-adrenaline is secreted in smaller quantities, making them want to overeat. Although tyrosine does have metabolic effects, you still have to do sufficient sustained physical exercise to burn off the fat or it will come back and refill the fat cells.

Tyrosine and exercise

Tyrosine is still not widely used, although it is not dangerous. The recommended dose is 500 to 1000 milligrams per day. Tyrosine is only effective as part of an appropriate diet and in combination with regular exercise. In these conditions, it is thought to accelerate the burning of fat and most of all it makes it possible to suppress the appetite (reducing it by 22% according to some research).

KEY FACTS

* Tyrosine is an amino acid which is thought to unblock the fats stored in the body.

* A tyrosine supplement suits people who are depressed and who tend to cope with stress by overeating.

51

repair the damage caused by childbirth

Childbirth is a harsh test for the stomach muscles. So you shouldn't just dive in thinking that intensive abdominal training is the right solution. First of all, work on the perineum.

What does the perineum do?

The perineum is a fasciculus of muscle attached like a hammock to the pelvis, the pubis and the sacrum. When it contracts, it holds in the urine, stools and gases. In order to do its job, the perineum must have good muscle tone. During pregnancy and childbirth it is put under a great deal of pressure and stretched to its limits. Before launching your flat stomach program at the gym, you must ensure that your perineum is capable of contracting. If not, the pressure of each muscle contraction will force the perineum to drop, ruining all your efforts to achieve a flat stomach.

The lift

Imagine that the perineum is a lift inside the body and that it can go up four floors to waist level. Contract your perineum, go up a floor, wait one second, then go up another floor. Continue in this way until you reach the fourth floor. Go back down to the first floor (not the ground floor!) before repeating the process again. Don't stiffen up and don't clench your buttocks.

The cross

This exercise is recommended by physiotherapists to regain the tone of the stomach muscles, perineum and buttocks. Lie down flat on your back, legs bent and arms crossed. Raise your pelvis for 5 seconds. Return to the start position, relax for 10 seconds and then start again. Repeat the exercise 10 times.

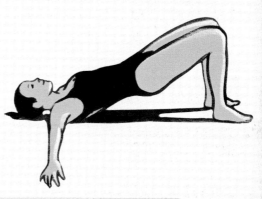

KEY FACTS

* You need to re-educate your perineum before starting your flat-stomach gym program.

* There can be no flat stomach with a weak perineum and a back that's too arched.

* After childbirth, 7 or 8 women out of 10 need to do this re-education.

52 check your hormonal balance

If you are aged 50 or over and getting symptoms such as hot flushes and sweats, you should have a review of your endocrine levels. A well-managed course of hormones could change your life.

Hormone replacement therapy is helpful for treatment of flushes and sweats, and dryness of the vagina as well as the prevention of osteoporosis and it may help with aching joints, fatigue and the general malaise some women feel during and after the menopause. However taking a course of HRT is not without its complications, including irregular bleeding, deep vein thrombosis and an increased risk of breast cancer and possibly heart disease and strokes. You really need to discuss this with your doctor.

Remember that many of the symptoms experienced by women in the menopause are often short-lived. Only a small proportion of women have hot flushes and sweats that persist for any length of time. HRT therapy is effective for moderate to severe hot flushes and sweats.

KEY FACTS

* If you are over 50 and are suffering troublesome symptoms of the menopause, arrange a consultation with your doctor.

* A hormone supplement suiting to your needs may enhance your sense of well-being.

53 Give your abs a daily workout

It takes will and determination, but the results will certainly make it all worthwhile... and quickly! Just ten or so minutes a day of abdominal exercises, whenever you like, but without a break, will make that difference.

Contract and relax There's no mystery to a flat stomach. You need to make it tight, firm and muscled. In order to obtain the optimum result, you need to alternate the contraction and stretching of the muscles. These phases of stretching should give you a real feeling of well being, but don't force it.

In practice Combine all the exercises described in this book and repeat several times in succession. Always start and finish in the position described for stretching the abdominal muscles: lie down flat on your back, arms together and straight out behind your head, and legs together and straight out. Your fingers and toes should continue the line of your body as if they wanted to keep on growing. Stretch for 5 to 8 seconds.

> Getting up without using your arms is often considered to be the best exercise for strengthening the abdominals, however this is untrue. The contraction of these muscles only allows the elevation of the body by about 30°.

> Moreover, you have to work on the hip muscles and place an unusual level of stress on the lower back, which could be dangerous.

KEY FACTS

* For visible results, you need to work on your abdominal muscles for several minutes a day.

* Alternate contractions and stretching.

54

get those lymphs circulating

A course of lymphatic drainage, administered by a qualified practitioner, is good for deep-down cleansing. It's vital if you know that you are clogged up with various toxins and if you tend to combine water retention and cellulite, both of which get in the way of your flat stomach goal.

Avoid bottlenecks

Lymph picks up the waste from our body and purifies it. The ganglions function like a miniature purification plant. Unfortunately, unlike the arterial blood, this white blood does not have the help of a heart to pump it around. Lymph circulates as best it can in the microscopic vessels but, if the neighbouring muscles do not contract, it stagnates. Avoid huge bottlenecks (and

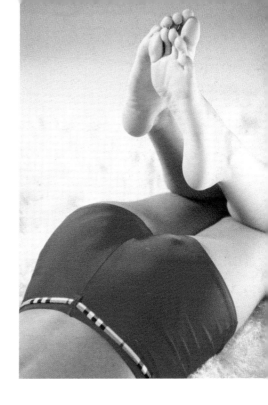

the creation of new cellulite dimpling), by making sure you take regular physical exercise and by following a course of manual lymphatic drainage.

Fifteen sessions for a good result

This type of massage has nothing in common with the pressure movements of muscular massage. It involves gentle, rhythmic hand movements that follow the lymphatic circuit to give it a boost. The physiotherapist starts with the ganglions located at the base of the neck, under the plexus and the armpits. Calm, relaxation and above all efficient drainage are the goals, and are dependant on you having about fifteen sessions close together.

for boosting the circulation without stress to the veins. Sports practised in water are good as they increase blood flow back from the legs to the heart and the output of urine by the kidneys – and as they are not weight-bearing, they are less stressful on the joints.

KEY FACTS

* Treat yourself to a course of lymphatic drainage sessions to boost your circulation.

* Officially, only physiotherapists can perform this massage.

* Try to commit to a walking programme to help the lymph and the blood to circulate.

55

find out about DHEA

DHEA is presently not available over the counter in some countries, including the UK. It has been shown to have undeniable anti-ageing properties – at least in tests on rodents and dogs. What is less widely known is that this hormone increases muscular mass at the expense of body fat.

DHEA: the mother of hormones

Studies on animals have shown that DHEA favours weight loss, even without a diet. However, it involves high doses that, applied to man, could have harmful effects. But even at the prescribed dose, DHEA still has an impact on excess weight, particularly in women who have stomachs distended by several pregnancies. A natural appetite suppressant, it melts the fat while at the same time increasing muscle production, with the calories being simply transformed into heat rather than stored.

No miracle cure

DHEA will only have an effect on you if, and only if, you really need it. And even if you do, don't expect a miracle. Some specialists consider the combination of a suitable diet, physical activity and DHEA as a winning formula, particularly in stabilizing weight, and a hormone supplement can act as a real boost for the disheartened. Dosage starts at 20 milligrams per day, rising to 75 milligrams or more, according to your needs. DHEA is available via the internet but has undergone no large-scale controlled trials, as in the case of HRT. It is likely that if the drug were used widely and regularly, unexpected side effects would occur, so you should accept that if you buy it you are treating yourself as a guinea pig.

> A DHEA supplement goes to make up the shortfall, but the hormone treatment must necessarily be monitored and its risks and benefits are still uncertain.

KEY FACTS

* Although DHEA is available on the internet, treatment is still controversial and you should consult your doctor if you think you need a DHEA supplement.

* DHEA is not recommended in cases of hormonal cancer.

56

You haven't paid much attention to what you eat until now and have never been inside a gym. But you're now blowing out 40 birthday candles and it's time to set in place a tummy-tackling programme.

prepare for the pre-menopause

Pick up good habits

On reaching the pre-menopause, women often complain of a prominent tummy... even the slim ones! Under the influence of hormones, the spine begins to shorten as the intervertebral discs dry out. Consequently, the stomach has to find space where it can, and in most cases this is in front. Since prevention is always easier than cure, particularly in this situaation, it's time to learn and to stick to some good habits that will allow you to limit this process.

Less sugar, more sport

Start by cutting out or cutting back on all foods made with refined sugar. Jams, cakes and other sweet things will cost you more and more dearly with regard to cellulite. And most importantly, get those trainers or sneakers out of the cupboard! You may work tirelessly on your abdominal muscles, but it's your whole body that you need to get moving. Not only is it the most effective way to maintain a slender figure, but it's also vital for conserving good, solid bones. Overall you will be firmer, stand up straighter and, hoorah, your tummy won't stick out.

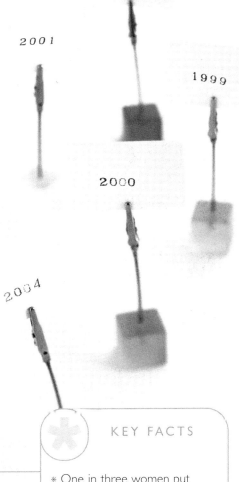

2001

1999

2000

2034

> After 40, take care. Restrict alcohol consumption to nights out with friends, cut back on fat and sugar and, most of all, take up a sport, if you haven't already.

57 learn about liposuction

Have you tried everything and your stomach still remains stubbornly flabby? Are you prepared to have surgery to get the result you want? Consult a plastic surgeon to find out if you are suitable for liposuction. This technique has developed a great deal and could present an acceptable solution.

Destroy the surplus fat! The process of liposuction is clear. It is not about reducing excess weight, but rather just minimizing localized excess fat deposits. Only around 20% of the fat is accessible to the surgeon. Liposuction aims to destroy the fat cells by removing them with the help of a tube introduced into the skin.

Weights and measures Be careful, liposuction is a proper surgical procedure. You should only consider it if you know you can control your diet, because we now know that new fatty deposits can form after the operation, and you will start storing fat again. After liposuction, you will have to use a compression bandage for several weeks.

● ● ● DID YOU KNOW?

> Liposuction was first introduced in 1977 by Fisher, who performed an internal 'milling' to destroy excess fatty tissues. In 1981 Fournier improved on the method with the tube.

> Average quantities of 1 to 1.5 litres (1¾ to 2½ pints) of fat are removed. The maximum is 3 litres (5 pints), and this limit should not be exceeded.

KEY FACTS

* Liposuction is used on localized deposits of excess fat, such as a flabby tummy.

* You can't have liposuction without also improving your diet and lifestyle.

58 seek the help of a surgeon

In certain cases, surgery may the last resort to rediscover your firm, flat, taut-skinned stomach. But you need to think seriously before launching yourself in this direction.

Abdominal plastic surgery If your efforts on a dietary and physical level have not yielded any result, if your hormonal balance is normal and your stomach still looks like a pouch, your last resort is an 'apronectomy' or abdominal plastic surgery. Under general anaesthetic, the surgeon takes away the excess skin, removes the excess fat and reforms the abdominal muscles to hold it all in.

Convalescence under surveillance This operation is advised for women who have had several children and cannot regain a 'normal' stomach. You will be in hospital for several days and need help at home afterwards as you will have trouble getting about. Lymphatic drainage sessions are essential during convalescence, which may last as long as a month, depending on the case.

KEY FACTS

* In certain specific cases, surgery can repair stomachs distended by pregnancies or unsuitable diets.

* Choose your surgeon carefully: this is an operation after all!

59

see the light!

As winter approaches, some people are very sensitive to the lack of sunlight. They actually develop a form of depression known as **SAD (Seasonal Affective Disorder)**, the results of which are an uncontrollable urge to snack and, consequently, a well-rounded tummy.

And the lights went out…

When sunlight is insufficient as it is in winter, changes occur in the neuro-transmitters in our brain, including a fall in the output of serotonin, a substance that suppresses our appetite. People who suffer from SAD have just two things in mind: sleeping and eating. Of course, it's not always to grated raw carrot that they turn, but more likely biscuits and chocolate. There are two solutions for this, a trip to the tropics

● ● ● D I D Y O U K N O W ?

> Nordic countries have long been familiar with seasonable depression and treat it with light therapy.

> Close to each of the Poles, the lack of sunlight lasts for six long months and those living there are often affected by a loss of energy, the need to sleep and an irresistible craving to eat sweet things.

to stock up on light or a phototherapy course. In the week following the start of the treatment, serotonin levels automatically increase and the appetite diminishes.

To the source

It's not about standing in front of spotlights or neon lighting in a nightclub. Phototherapy, much used in hospitals, faithfully reproduces the spectrum of sunlight. To achieve this it must reach 2,500 lux or the equivalent to 5 times the light of a brightly lit office (a living room may be only 100 lux). These lights have long been used as aquarium equipment, but now you can buy special light bulbs or even phototherapy equipment to use at home. A light treatment with an hour of exposure a day should be enough to get you through winter (1-2 hours/day, up to 4 hours starting in autumn and daily in winter).

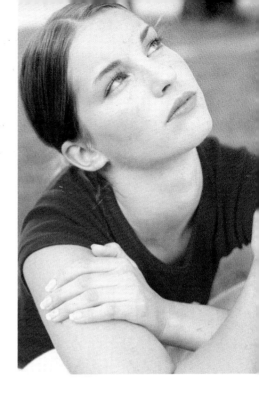

> We now use phototherapy with great success. But it only works by using the full light spectrum which can be seen in the rainbow, while traditional light bulbs, which are not complete, only reproduce the waves represented by the red-orange.

KEY FACTS

∗ Light therapy is accepted as an effective treatment for seasonal depression.

∗ It is recommended by the American Psychiatric Association and there are various self-help organizations, including SADA in the UK.

60 get yourself a personal trainer

A personal trainer is the solution chosen by numerous celebrities to stay in shape and keep their figure. It's an idea that's gaining ground and is not out of reach, particularly if you team up with a friend.

Your advice, your personality, your progress If your stomach needs a complete overhaul and you haven't done any work on it for years, a personalized program may prove very useful. All the more so if you have certain weaknesses, such as weak tendons or back pain. You can either seek the advice of a trained physiotherapist who will show you the exercises you need to do, or you can employ the services of a sports trainer.

Hello! Is my trainer there? The majority of gyms now offer 'personalized monitoring' with a sports advisor permanently available. In some of then you can benefit from solo sessions with this expert. But of course you can also have the trainer come to your home, to design an exercise program that is just right for you.

● ● ● DID YOU KNOW?

> The coaching formula is so much in vogue nowadays that some gyms only offer this service.

> It can be expensive so why not find a friend to share the costs with you? You can motivate each other and have fun at the same time as getting fit!

KEY FACTS

* Nothing beats a personal trainer for giving your muscles a really good workout.

* A personal trainer will devise a program especially tailored for you that will help to get back that flat stomach.

case study

(from France)

DHEA helped me to lose my stomach!

«Since the menopause started, I continued doing all my intensive physical activity but I couldn't get rid of my stomach. I did all sorts of sports and followed lifestyle advice on staying in shape. My doctor advised me to try DHEA, explaining to me that since my problem was caused by hormones, maybe it had a hormonal solution. Since I've been taking it, I've lost some weight and I feel that my physical activity is much more effective. I feel better and my libido is much higher. But in addition to taking any hormone replacement or DHEA, it is important to improve your lifestyle. There's a whole series of things to do to feel better. In all events, as a very sporty person, I think that I recover more quickly and I'm less susceptible to infections. I'm not shattered by 11pm anymore.»

useful addresses

» Homeopathy

British Homeopathic Association
Hahnemann House
29 Park Street West
Luton LU1 3BE
tel: 0870 444 3950

The Society of Homeopaths
4a Artizan Road
Northampton NN1 4HU
tel: 01604 621400

Australian Homeopathic Association
PO Box 430, Hastings
Victoria 3915
Australia
www.homeopathyoz.org

» Herbal medicine

British Herbal Medicine Association
Sun House
Church Street
Stroud, Gloucester GL5 1JL
tel: 01453 751389

National Institute of Medical Herbalists
56 Longbrook Street
Exeter, Devon EX4 6AH
tel: 01392 426022

» Massage

British Massage Therapy Council
www.bmtc.co.uk

Association of British Massage Therapists
42 Catharine Street
Cambridge CB1 3AW
tel: 01223 240 815

European Institute of Massage
42 Moreton Street
London SW1V 2PB
tel: 020 7931 9862

» Menopause

British Menopause Society
www.the-bms.org

National Osteoporosis Society
Camerton, Bath BA2 0PJ
tel: 01761 471771
www.nos.org.uk

International Osteoporosis Foundation
www.osteofound.org

North America Menopause Society
PO Box 94527, Cleveland
Ohio 44101-4527, USA

Australasian Menopause Society
PO Box 1228, Buderim
Queensland 4556
Australia

» Qi Gong

Qi Gong Association of America
PO Box 252
Lakeland, MN, USA
email: info@nqa.org

» Relaxation therapy

British Autogenic Society
The Royal London
Homoeopathic Hospital
Greenwell Street
London W1W 5BP

British Complementary Medicine Association
PO Box 5122
Bournemouth BH8 0WG
tel: 0845 345 5977

» SAD (Seasonal Affective Disorder)

SAD Association
PO Box 989
Steyning BN44 3HG
www.sada.org.uk

acknowledgements

Cover: B. Shearer/Option Photo; p. 9: O. Graf/Zefa; p. 11: M. Möllenberg/Zefa; p. 12-13: M. Möllenberg/Zefa; p. 17, 33, 35, 40, 43, 45, 63, 65, 73, 81, 91, 92, 117: Neo Vision/Photonica; p. 19: Holz/Zefa; p. 23: H. Winkler/Zefa; p. 25: © Akiko Ida; p. 29: E. Mc Connell/Pix; p. 31: M. Thomsen/Zefa; p. 37: T. Hoenig/Zefa; p. 39: Per Magnus Persson/Photonica; p. 47: p. Verdi/option Photo; p. 51: Pinto/Zefa; p. 53: Emely/Zefa; p. 55: Gulliver/Zefa; p. 57: Miles/Zefa; p. 59: Emely/Zefa; p. 66: R. Daly/Stone; p. 71: © Akiko Ida; p. 75: Gulliver/Zefa; p. 76-77: Star/Zefa; p. 83: G. Girardot/Marie Claire; p. 84: Emely/Zefa; p. 88-89: Pinto/Zefa; p. 95: © Akiko Ida; p. 105: M. Möllenberg/Zefa; p. 107: Miles/Zefa; p. 113: Miles/Zefa; p. 121: M. Möllenberg/Zefa.

Illustrations: Marianne Maury Kaufmann pages 14-15, 26-27, 60-61, 98-99, 102-103 and 108-109.

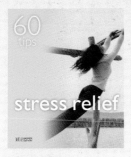

stress relief

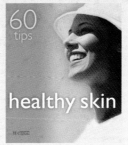

healthy skin

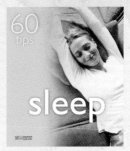

sleep

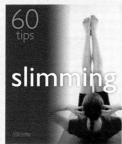

slimming

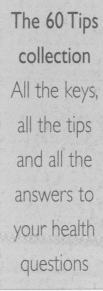

The 60 Tips collection

All the keys, all the tips and all the answers to your health questions

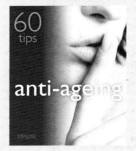

anti-ageing

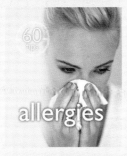

allergies

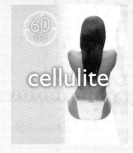

cellulite

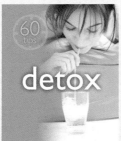

detox

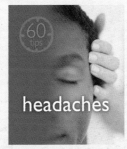

headaches

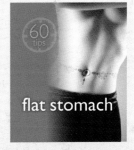

flat stomach

Editorial directors: Caroline Rolland and Delphine Kopff

Editorial assistant: Marine Barbier

Graphic design: Guylaine Moi

Layout: G & C MOI

Final checking: Fabienne Hélou

Illustrations: Alexandra Bentz and Guylaine Moi

Production: Felicity O'Connor

Translation: JMS Books LLP

© Hachette Livre (Hachette Pratique) 2002
This edition published in 2005 by Hachette Illustrated UK, Octopus Publishing Group Ltd.,
2–4 Heron Quays, London E14 4JP

English translation by JMS Books LLP (email: moseleystrachan@blueyonder.co.uk)
Translation © Octopus Publishing Group Ltd.

A CIP catalogue for this book is available from the British Library

ISBN-13: 978-1-84430-091-4

ISBN-10: 1-84430-091-9

Printed in Singapore by Tien Wah Press